Taboo Sex Stories:

Erotica Seductive Sex Fantasies for Adults. Threesome, GangBang, BDSM and Femdom

the rendering of legal, financial, medical or professional advice. The content within this book has been derived from various sources. Please consult a licensed professional before attempting any techniques outlined in this book.

By reading this document, the reader agrees that under no circumstances is the author responsible for any losses, direct or indirect, which are incurred as a result of the use of information contained within this document, including, but not limited to, — errors, omissions, or inaccuracies.

Table of Contents

Blind Pleasure

Catherine, a hesitant wife, gives in to Rich, her husband's greatest fantasy: He wants to see her fucked by other men. Yes, men—as in plural. He wants to watch her gangbanged while he enjoys watching every single moment of it, but she's not so convinced. She is nervous about what to expect but soon finds that she doesn't have to be so afraid of what is to cum, over and over again. She goes off to the local swinger's club with him for a night she will never forget—and may even want to repeat some time.

"Catherine."

The sound of my husband's voice sent a shiver down my spine, and the skin on my arms began to prickle into goosebumps. I knew what he wanted. I kept my eyes planted firmly on my reflection as I finished getting myself ready to his standards. Eyeliner, heavy and winged into the perfect cat-eye. Black, smoky shadow was blended onto my eyelids. My eyes, the most indistinctive shade of flat brown, looked bigger, and I could see my own hesitation in them.

"Catie."

His voice was quieter and more urgent. More needing. I felt his hand on the small of my back, and it sent a quick shock shooting within me. I loved his touch—I couldn't deny that. It was everyone else's that I was hesitant about.

5

Still, I kept my gaze planted on myself, putting the finishing touches on my face. My lips, a deep pink, almost red against my naturally pale skin. My brown hair was straightened and lay almost pin-straight down to my shoulders, curving in just slightly toward my cheeks to frame my narrow face.

"It's time."

His hand slid off of my back, leaving the place that he had touched, feeling almost uncomfortably cold, vying for his touch again. His fingers wrapped around my wrist and pulled, beckoning me to turn, and I did to look at him.

My husband, Rich, was conventionally attractive. Between the two of us, he blew me out of the water. He had a perfectly sculpted jawline, strong and masculine, with just a hint of 5-o-clock shadow across it, and a strong brow. His eyes were bright blue and his hair, almost black and trimmed to create a taper cut. He was wearing a tight, black t-shirt and a pair of tight jeans that betrayed his large bulge in his pants. I looked over him and couldn't help it. Just the sight of him, all ready to go was enough to make me wet. He smirked at me as I looked him over, satisfied.

He grabbed my hand and took me outdoors to the car. We drove in a heavy silence to the club we were going to. We had never done anything

6

like this before, and while I had agreed to do so, it was more because he wanted to than anything else. He wanted to see other men fuck me; he had said one day when we were showering after a night of X-rated passion. His cock had quickly hardened at the suggestion as he watched me, slowly washing away the sweat from the night. I had agreed to do it for him, but I couldn't say that I was particularly excited about it.

"You'll change your tune real quick, hon," he had replied when I shrugged my shoulders. "Think of all the men that are there—to please *you*. They're there to have fun with you." And so, here we were, preparing to enter a swinger's club for the first time. Rich had figured everything out on his own; he arranged for the night, for the reservations that we apparently needed, and for the people that would be there.

Before I knew it, we were parked outside of a nondescript building. I never would have guessed that inside was a club, apparently full of people that wanted to trade partners. It looked like a simple brick building without a sign, and if it weren't for the cars parked all over it or the fact that I saw another couple entering the building, I'd have assumed we were in the wrong place. I was expecting something a bit... More flashy? This was certainly not.

Rich squeezed my hand and brought me back to reality. I turned to look at him and was immediately met with his lips on mine. His tongue danced over my bottom lip, waiting for me to open mine, and I quickly obliged, feeling his tongue against mine. His hand slid up my arm and to my breast, giving it a quick squeeze. When he came up for air, breaking the kiss, he smirked at me again. God, I loved that smirk. "Don't sweat it, hon. You're going to love it; I know you will." He kept massaging my breast, playing with it, but this time, he let his finger linger over my nipple, pressing in.

I gasped, feeling myself begin to get wet, and my clit twitched, beginning to swell, and I leaned in for another kiss. My hand snaked around to feel his cock, so big in his pants and so trapped that I just *had* to free them from their cage. I unbuttoned the pants and undid the zipper, reaching in to pull it out. It was at full attention and ready to go. My hand ran over it, and I felt his body tense as he moaned against my lips. This time, it was my turn to smirk as I slowly rubbed his cock, up and down. Up and down.

He reached down to touch my pussy, slipping underneath my little black dress and right past the little black thong that I had worn to match, his fingers expertly finding my clit. He rubbed on it, and my legs spread open for him, granting full access. I ran my hand over his cock, feeling the shaft get harder. The car

8

smelled of our passion as I quickly undid my seatbelt and leaned over to take him in my mouth, but he protested, quickly pulling his hand away from me and leaving me wanting.

"Slow down," he said with a dark chuckle. He was watching me with amusement as he took his fingers into his mouth, sucking off every bit of liquid that I had left on him. "We have plenty of time for that later."

So off we went, into the club, and we picked up a few shots, followed by a cocktail each, on our way, to "ease our nerves," Rich had said, but I knew he just meant mine. I was watching the way that his clothes clung to his body, and especially to his crotch, watching that bulge that remained there. No one batted an eye as we walked through the club. There was music, low, pulsing, but nondescript in the background to fill any silence, and couples and groups were talking quietly amongst each other as they sipped their drinks and looked at each other like chunks of meat. It almost made me nervous until I realized that I was looking at my husband in exactly the same way. With our drinks in hand, my husband led me to a private room in the back. When we entered, I saw that it was decorated like a hotel suite; there was a bathroom connected to it and a queen-sized poster bed.

The lighting was dim, and I finished my drink, placing the drink on a nightstand. The alcohol left me pleasantly buzzed, and Rich grinned. He could see the flush on my cheeks, even in the absence of light. He made his way over to me and roughly pushed me onto the bed, gripping at my breasts with both hands for a moment before they both slipped into the top of my dress, His fingers pinched at my nipples, delicately at first and then with more fervor as he nibbled at my neck before slamming his lips against mine. I could taste the alcohol on his breath and it just made me want him more. I spread my legs and thrust my hips against his, rubbing myself on his hard cock. I reached my hands down to undo his pants, but he stopped me, grabbing my wrist and then attaching a strap around them. I stopped, blinking in surprise. We had played with the restraints every now and then at home and I recognized them as the ones that we used. The restraint went around one of the posts on the bed and then another came out for the other hand.

Before I could protest, he had pulled out a pocket vibrator, placing it against my clit first and then teasing the slit of my pussy. My hips bucked upwards at the jolt, and a moan escaped my lips. He left it there as he placed a tie around each of my ankles as well, leaving me spread-eagle on the bed. I was enjoying the vibrator so much that I hardly noticed.

He reached back up for the vibrator, taking it slowly from its position and back up to my clit and then turned it off just as I was really starting to get into it. I could feel myself starting to drip, and I was certain that I had already left a wet spot on the bed. Before I could beg for more, I felt Rich's lips kissing me. His tongue flicked across my clit, making me gasp and shudder. He licked with a bit more force, one hand snaking up to grasp my chest. He pinched and pulled at my nipple as he licked, his tongue expertly tracing my clit until he moved downward, licking at my opening as well. He let his tongue tease the entrance just a bit longer with a quick "Mmm..." against me.

"Rich, fuck me," I managed to moan out as I felt my body flex. I tried to reach down to grab his head, but the restraints held me back. I felt him laugh against me. I was desperate to get that cock inside me, and he knew it. He knew how much I longed for it. He climbed atop me in the bed and pressed himself against me. He smelled like me, a faint, almost pungent scent, and he looked down at me. I leaned up to rub against him some more, but he pulled away.

"Oh, believe me, you'll be fucked plenty," he practically purred as he pulled something else out of his pocket. It was a black blindfold, and it was very quickly wrapped around my head. I couldn't see anything, and for a moment, I felt a hint of anxiety, but that was quickly forgotten when I heard a zip and felt his cock enter me.

It was slow at first, just the tip, and immediately, my body tensed up in pleasure. I felt every inch of him as he slid into me, and I squeezed against him, moaning softly. I tried to reach out for him, but my hands were restrained. "Good girl," he said softly as he thrust harder and harder. His balls bounced against my ass, sounding like slaps, and my pussy got even wetter than I thought was possible. I felt his hands clawing at my chest as if trying to tear away the dress that I was wearing. The restraints held me back, and it was almost hotter that I couldn't see what was happening. I was in total ecstasy as he rammed into me and I heard him grunt in equal pleasure.

"Fuck me harder, Rich," I moaned out, and he obliged, but just as I was about to orgasm, he stopped and pulled away. I was left in shock and utter silence. "... Rich?" I called out, only to hear him chuckling from across the room.

"Have fun," he said, and then I knew it was beginning.

Within seconds, I could smell a new man near me; he smelled of aftershave, woody almost. My heart was pounding in my chest, and I was almost afraid to speak when I realized what was about to happen, but all apprehension melted away as soon as I felt another vibrator rubbing against my clit as a finger slipped into my pussy.

"Mmm... Nice, wet, and tight," the voice said, almost breathy as the man that I couldn't see felt me up. He felt good. Maybe it was the alcohol and lack of inhibition, or the fact that Rich had been driving me crazy all night, or the fact that I had complete permission to fuck a strange man with him watching, but those first seconds were better than I expected.

Before I could say a word, I felt his fingers probe into me again, holding the vibrator in place with what I assume was his palm as his other hand squeezed my ass, pulling at my cheeks. His fingers teased my asshole, and my entire body tightened up in pleasure. I moaned as the vibrator was replaced with a face that felt clean-shaven—there was none of the prickling I usually felt with Rich. I felt him sucking, kissing, and licking at my clit, slowly at first, tantalizingly teasing me. "Such a bad little girl, look how much she wants it," he murmured between my lips. The feeling sent shivers down my spine. "Do you want it, you hot little slut?"

I moaned again, practically unable to speak as he continued to suck away. I felt him pull away and heard another zip as he undid his pants and the rustling of clothing. His cock felt different—it was wider than Rich's as it rubbed at my slit, teasing my swollen lips as he did so. I thrust my hips up, trying to get him to enter, but he pulled back, laughing. "She's ready to go, Rich!" he called out, and I heard Rich chuckling. I could hear the pleasure in his

13

voice—it was low and almost urgent. He was enjoying every moment of this, so why shouldn't I?

I heard footsteps approach me as the strange man's cock continued to tease me, moving up and down, sometimes, sliding across my clit and sometimes circling my asshole, leaving me breathless with anticipation. My senses were on overdrive; I could hear his own breathing change as he enjoyed himself as well. Suddenly, I felt a mouth on my neck, and I smelled another scent—this one was citrusy.

"She's definitely a looker, isn't she?" said another voice, and I felt his hands lightly brushing over my arms. I shivered at the touch, moaning as the first man, the one who smelled of sandalwood, finally thrust into me. His cock was longer than Rich's too, it felt like, as it slid deeper and deeper, slowly penetrating me until I felt his balls against my ass. He held it there as I felt the other man pull down my dress, leaving my breasts bare. I knew my nipples were perfectly erect at that point, and I could feel a faint breeze over them. It was warm. Was it his breath? His head must have been awfully close to them, and citrus man gently touched each one. Then, he pinched a bit harder, leaving me moaning again. I couldn't do anything; I was stuck exactly in place, but I really just wanted to ride the cock that was inside of me.

I felt the man who was next to me lower his head down to take my nipple into my mouth, and he bit down on it, hard enough to send a shiver down my spine but not so hard to hurt. The cock that was in me thrust harder, and I cried out, but not in pain. I felt the man inside of me squeeze at my ass and then suddenly smack it hard enough to sting. I cried out but felt myself get wetter against him, and I clenched against every inch of his girth, feeling it fill me. His cock pulsated against me as he pulled it out, never quite all the way, before slamming back into me, all the while I felt the man's fingers clawing at my ass more and more.

"I want more," I managed to gasp out, and in response, I got another slap across the ass, a bit more forceful this time, and I yelped in response. This brought another slap quickly, followed by another.

"You want more, you little slut?" Sandalwood said, his breath starting to hitch as he kept slamming into me. I moaned in response as I felt another slap. I'm sure my ass was red by that point, but I was too lost in passion to care. "Yes, please give me more," I managed to moan out between breaths.

Then, I felt another hand on me suddenly. This hand was different. It was rougher. Stronger. More confident as it caressed over my body. Three. There were three pairs of hands on me

15

now, and strangely, I didn't mind. In fact, I loved every moment of it. One pair held me in place as Sandalwood continued to thrust with as much force as he could muster, and I lifted my hips so that my clit would rub against his pelvis. Citrus continued to knead and suck at my breasts and nipples, and this new pair of hands was slowly exploring my body with his hands. I heard more zipping, and very quickly, a rock-hard cock was shoved in my face.

"Open," I heard a gruff voice command, and I did so, turning my head toward him. He shoved himself into my mouth so hard that I gagged at first, tears springing to my eyes. I let my tongue roll over his dick, lingering on the frenulum before pushing it deeper into my mouth.

I could hardly take it. Every nerve in my body felt like it was on overdrive as I was pleasured from three different men, and I could hear my husband's own breathing, almost ragged in the corner. Was he jerking himself as he watched? The thought of Rich's face, enjoying watching his wife become a toy for all of these men, was enough for me, but he loved it.

I knew I wasn't going to be able to last much longer. I could feel my own pleasure building and building until I could hardly take it anymore. My own moans had grown louder, and I could feel my body taking control, moving and grinding into Sandalwood harder and harder. Citrus was sucking harder than before, so hard that it would have hurt, but in the moment, I loved it.

Right as I was about to cum, I felt Sandalwood pull his dick out of me and leave me thrusting my body upward, searching blindly for him. He wasn't there, but I could hear him chucking. I could feel the warmth of his body radiating off of him, just outside of my reach.

"Beg for it," he said.

My mouth was full of another cock, licking and sucking on it, and I whined. I tried to open my mouth to pull away to speak, but the man held me in place roughly, twisting his hand in my hair to keep me right where I was. I got it then—I wasn't going to be allowed to finish until they were each satisfied. I sucked on his dick with as much passion as I could muster. I could feel his shaft twitching and bulging in my mouth as I continued to slurp at it. He held me in place and slammed himself into my mouth, letting himself go down my throat to make me gag. He didn't let up, going harder and harder until I tasted him. The salty, hot liquid shot down my throat, burning and making me gag as I felt him cum into my mouth. His cock twitched and pulsated in my mouth as he held me there to his own pleasure, and when he pulled out, I moved to spit, but he held my mouth shut.
"Swallow it," he told me. I did, shuddering as it went down my throat, leaving its aftertaste in

my mouth. I wasn't normally a swallower, but nothing about this situation was normal. It was strangely erotic to be ordered around, and at this point, I think it would have been impossible for me to get any wetter. I could feel my own juices dribbling down to my ass as I was spread out, and the sheets right underneath me were soaked. The whole room smelled musty, of sex and men, and I *loved* it.

"Please," I said breathlessly, thrusting my pelvis up, looking for Sandalwood. He had to have been there somewhere. But then, another dick was shoved in my face. I sucked it in greedily and tasted myself all over it, and that woody smell of the man who had, only moments prior, been thrusting into me was standing over me. He shuddered as my lips wrapped around his shaft, licking myself up and savoring the taste. He was so hard, and he was so wide that my jaw was opened up almost uncomfortably far as I took him in, gently, slowly, sensually using my tongue to caress his head and shaft.

Then, I felt something else beneath me. Was that Citrus? I couldn't smell him near me anymore, I realized, and that must have been why. He was underneath me now, rubbing his own cock against me. He started up on my clit, making me moan against Sandalwood's dick as he did. It was a gentle touch, but it was enough to drive me crazy with desire. I wanted him, and I wanted him *then*.

I thrust my hips up just right, taking the cock into my body as I continued to suck on the first one. I groaned in ecstasy as I felt the length of him enter me. He pulled my legs up as much as he could with the constraints and thrust his way into me as hard as he could. I cried out, only to have my head thrust back onto the cock in my mouth, and I continued to suck on it.

Citrus was a much more sensual fucker than Sandalwood had been. He entered me and gyrated his hips, allowing himself to touch more of me. He angled himself just right to shoot toward the top of my vagina, rubbing against the walls and leaving me hotter than before. As my body got closer, and I felt more of my own wetness dribble out and down onto Citrus, I felt him pull away, just like before. I wanted him so badly, but I knew what was happening. I needed to finish off Sandalwood first.

I sucked on Sandalwood harder, craning my neck as far as I could until he pushed himself toward me. My nose was against his groin. It was unshaven; I could feel the hairs tickling against my face as I took as much of him in as I could, letting my lips tighten around him before pulling away. "That's right, you little slut," he managed to hiss out as I pulled away, letting the tip of my tongue trace along his shaft as I did it. I smiled until the next thrust from Citrus made me moan, almost losing myself in the pleasure. Sandalwood's hand, yanking my hair, brought me back to reality, and I repeated that motion, again and again, getting quicker and quicker until he was shaking. I teased his head with my tongue. I could feel his dick getting firmer. He was getting close, and I could taste the precum on the tip as I flicked it with my tongue. I shoved him down my throat as hard as I could manage without gagging and sucked, and then I felt him jolt, thrusting himself into my mouth as again, I was rewarded with the taste of cum shooting down my throat. His was slightly less pungent than the first man's, and I sucked it down greedily, licking along his shaft as his body continued to be rocked with enjoyment. I grinned. Mission accomplished. Now, there was nothing standing in my way.

Citrus slammed deeper than before into my body, and I felt his weight atop me as he climbed into the position that he wanted. I could smell him as he fucked me, and I moaned out, craning my head to kiss him as he continued to slam into me. I was searching for him, yearning for his mouth, but before I could find it, it was back on my nipple, flicking it with his tongue, sending my whole body convulsing. I was so close. "Fuck me harder," I managed to whisper between gasping breaths, my mouth now gloriously free from cock as I leaned up, placing my head into the crook of his neck.

He obliged instantly, shoving his dick harder into my body, and I lost myself in the moment. I cried out and rubbed myself against his pelvis as he continued to thrust, and almost immediately, all of the frustration and tension was released in ecstasy as I *finally* got the orgasm I had been waiting for. I felt my pussy clench around his dick harder and harder as he thrust, cumming within me to the feeling of my walls tightening. It was so intense that I lost myself, unaware of everything in that instant. I collapsed against the bed; all energy thoroughly drained from my body. I couldn't keep going even if I wanted to.

When I regained my wits, I realized it was almost silent, but I could hear someone shuffling around. I sat there in my post-sex haze, utterly exhausted and uninterested in what was going on around me, and I suddenly felt the restraints loosen and fall off and then felt my blindfold removed.

The room was surprisingly empty. I could see Rich staring at me with a look of arousal, admiration, and satisfaction all in one. He was thrilled to have seen me do what I had done. I was totally exhausted on the bed, and even freed up, I was not sure that I wanted to get up and do anything.

Rich smirked at me as I laid there in my post-sex high. "You ready for another round?" he murmured, running his hand up and down my body, sending a shiver down my spine.

I laughed as he got on top of me to kiss me unabashedly, his tongue dancing in my mouth as he savored the taste of others on my lips. His own cock was pressed against me, bare and rubbing against my thoroughly fucked, swollen pussy. I kissed him back. Surely, round two wouldn't be so bad. It was the least I could do to repay him for the fun I had.

Variety Is the Spice of Sex

Lindsey loved fucking new people. For her, fucking was something exciting and new, and while she loved fucking her husband, she wanted more. She wanted the act of exploring new bodies and getting new sensations and new connections. Her husband, Matt, has always seemed uninterested in the threesome or open relationship life, but for his wife, he's willing to try anything once. They open up a to their neighbor, sexy Delilah for some threesome fun to try to accommodate Lindsey's needs, and spend a day fucking harder than they have ever fucked before, leaving both Matt and Lindsey thoroughly satisfied.

I was bored.

I was being fucked by my husband, but I was completely bored out of my mind. Sex had grown dull. Sure, we could bring in toys. We did that a lot—I had toys of every kind imaginable. Rabbit vibes and cock rings and dildos galore, but none of them could keep my attention for very long at all. I wanted *more*. I wanted something else that would keep me happy. I wasn't sure what I wanted yet, but I knew that whatever it was, it wasn't this.

I pinched and kneaded at my nipples as my husband fucked me from behind. He grunted and groaned and unleaded within my pussy, collapsing onto me as he did. I could feel his heart pounding in his chest as he rested there for a moment before he turned his head to kiss me. He smiled at me, but it quickly faltered. "Again?" Matt asked with a hesitant frown.

I averted my gaze, almost ashamed that I was unable to enjoy the moment. We had tried everything that I could think of. We had done some of that teacher-student roleplay. It wasn't for me. We tried some light bondage, but I didn't care for that, either. I was just *bored*. This was the first relationship that I had been in for longer than a few months, and I almost thought that what I needed was something fresh. Fresh meat to enjoy or something. It was exciting to explore new bodies sometimes, and I felt like I hadn't been able to do that. I loved my husband, sure, but sexually? I was an explorer. I wanted to get out, fuck my brains out, and fuck as many people as I could. I had given up that life when I got married, but a part of me couldn't help but think that that was what I was missing.

"Is there anything I can do?" asked Matt.

I shook my head. It would be another night for the vibe in the bath with a glass of wine for me. I didn't need to make him feel worse or more inadequate about it.

"Do you want to fuck other people?" he finally asked me. I could hear it in his voice. It was almost breaking him to suggest it, but he loved me, and he wanted me to be happy.

I hesitated, but he must have seen the excitement that I tried to hide in my face. I saw his shoulders fall.

"What about a threesome?" I suggested suddenly.

He looked at me, confused.

"I don't want to fuck someone on my own," I told him. "I want you to join in. Wouldn't you want another toy to play with?" I winked at him and slapped his ass, enjoying the quick bounce as I did, squeezing and kneading the muscle. His ass was firmly toned. He, for one, did not skip leg day, that was for sure.

Matt sighed. "Lindsey, I don't know..." He looked at me with mixed emotions swirling in his green eyes.

"You'll love it," I promised him, giving him a quick kiss and nibbling on his lip. "It's fun."

He shrugged his shoulders. I was his only partner that he had ever had; he had wanted to save himself for marriage. He wasn't religious or anything, but he hadn't wanted to, shall we say, play the field; he wanted to keep sex something special for himself. But let's be real—a quick fuck is so much fun.

I grinned. "Trust me?"

He sighed again and nodded his head. "But no dicks. I'm firm on that one."

"Fine by me!" I said with a grin. I slapped his ass again, giggling as it bounced. There was a pink print on his cheek now as I clenched. I saw dick start to harden again as I did it, and I smiled at him, genuinely excited. I pulled him forward, kissing him, and he kissed back, ready for round two.

I did all of the work from that point on. I screened out options that would be interested in a bit of rough fun with us. I looked for women only, knowing Matt's stance, and I didn't mind myself. Sometimes, all you want is an extra pair of tits to fondle that aren't your own. Eventually, I had found the perfect person: The young neighbor that had just moved into the apartment next door.

Delilah was a perky, young 19 years old. Perfect tits, double-Ds on her hourglass figure. Her skin was a deep olive color, and her hair was down to her waist, black, thick, and I could only imagine pulling it myself as I played with those perfect little nipples that I made sure to check out and sample before choosing her to be the perfect partner. She was *gorgeous*. She was kinky, too—she had shown me her collection of restraints and even a few leather floggers, and I knew that we would be in for fun.

She knocked at the door, and when I opened it, she looked shy; she was almost too nervous to enter. I grabbed her wrist brusquely, immediately feeling a thrill as I pulled her in. This would be fun, and I was determined to enjoy each and every moment of it. The thought of a fresh, new body made me wet; I could feel my pussy twitch as I led her in. She looked at Matt and blushed a bit, but it just made me want her more.

Matt was sitting on our bed, naked and almost lazily stroking his own cock, displaying it for Delilah to see. He seemed a bit hesitant but was willing to give it a shot.

I took off my robe that I had been wearing to open the door, revealing that I was perfectly naked underneath and looked at Delilah. She was eyeing my husband's cock with a mixture of being impressed and desiring to get her own hands on it. I could see that look in her eyes— the look of lust. The look of her lips parting slightly as she inhaled. The shine of her eyes dilating as she looked at him. She wanted him, and that was enough to make me happy.

"You ready?" I purred as I reached over to pull Delilah's shirt over her head. She nodded her head and turned her eyes to me, taking in every inch of my body. I instinctively straightened out, pushing my chest outward more, and Delilah reached up to grab them. She ran her fingers over my nipples, pinching and rubbing at them, and I gasped at the feeling. Her fingers were so soft and warm as they worked their magic, the touch of a woman who was clearly experienced with the female body.

I leaned in to kiss Delilah, watching Matt's reaction as I did. He watched us intently, and I could see the way his cock twitched when I did it. I smiled against Delilah's lips as my tongue parted them and made its way into her mouth, tasting her. She tasted sweet, almost like a cup of wine. Had she had to drink a glass of wine to loosen up? I chuckled as I nibbled on her lips, and I led her to bed to join Matt.

Matt grinned as we did and opened his arms to us. I settled in on the left side of him, and Delilah was on the right. I pulled her in again to kiss, both of our breasts resting against Matt's chest as we did so. I moaned as I kissed her, and I felt Matt reach up to grab my breast and touch it. He touched my nipples with his own fingers. They were rougher than Delilah's; I immediately noticed. He flicked his fingers over them and was just a bit tougher than I was.

I reached down for Matt's hand on my breast and removed it, guiding it over to feel Delilah's as well, and I immediately felt him tense up, his breathing picking up. Then, I pulled away from

Delilah's lips, pushing her down to kiss Matt as well.

He reciprocated, his cock twitching as he did. I reached down to stroke it, running my nails gently up and down the shaft, making him shudder as he continued to kiss Delilah, with more fervor as I continued to play with him. He bit her lip, and I could hear him groan as I lowered my head down to lick him. I used just my tongue at first, running it up and down just as I had done with my nails. I saw his hips shift upward as he sought out my mouth, or any other wet hole he could get his cock in, and I obliged, taking it between my lips and hearing him moan against Delilah. After all, this had to be just as enjoyable, if not more so, for him than for me if I wanted him to feel like he wanted to do this again. I was in for the long haul, and I didn't mind sharing my new toy. I turned to look at Delilah, who was shifting to straddle him now, his hand both reaching for her breasts, kneading, tugging, and rubbing them between his hands. I could smell her wetness between her legs as she continued to kiss him, and I shifted down a bit to let her make her way downward. I pulled her hips, guiding her perfectly round ass down to him. I lined her up and took Matt's cock, still wet with my saliva, and put it into her. As soon as it felt her lips, it thrust upwards, and she moaned, throwing her head back.

Then, he thrust again and again. He was watching her intently, watching those perfect breasts bouncing on her chest, nipples pointed out, and still shimmering with saliva. He turned his attention back to me then and reached out with his hand to grasp my breasts as well. Mine were just as big, but age had already started to weigh them down. He didn't seem to mind as he greedily tugged and squeezed at them. His fingers glossed over my nipples, and I felt myself get wetter, my own clit starting to swell in anticipation of my turn for fun.

I watched as Delilah rode Matt harder and harder. She started to really moan and whine. "Oh, Matt!" she groaned, her head thrown back. "Fuck me harder!"

I slapped her ass, seeing the red mark appear almost immediately, but she only moaned louder. I grinned and slapped her again and again. I could feel myself starting to drip down my legs as they continued to fuck, and before they could get too into it, I interrupted the fun. I pulled Delilah up and off of Matt, pushing her down next to him. She gasped, looking up at me, almost in surprise. I could see the wetness from their fucking glistening between her thighs. Her pussy was perfectly waxed and hair-free. Perfect.

I looked over my new toy and forced her legs open. She was caught off guard, but she obliged, and I quickly buried my face between her lips, feeling that one little nub that seemed so hard for so many men to find. She gasped and shuddered as my tongue ran over her. I positioned myself just right on my knees, head down, and ass raised. Matt watched as I continued to lick at Delilah and seemed to get the idea as I shifted. He could enter from behind.

Matt quickly got into position and slammed into me quickly. "Lindsey, you're so wet," he groaned as he slid all the way, stopping only when his balls slapped my ass. I chuckled at him as I continued to lick Delilah's clit, feeling her shift at the feeling. She moaned as she continued to get licked. As I felt her getting closer to cumming, I slapped her ass suddenly. It surprised her, judging by the yelp, but judging by the gush of fluids in my face, she loved it. I slapped her again and reached up to take her breast in my hand.

Matt continued to fuck me from behind, and I kept my composure, sucking on that little nub. I slide my fingers into Delilah, one at first, then another. Then, I angle them just right, reaching around to get to that magical g-spot, and as soon as I reach it, I hear her moan, her hips shooting up as soon as I touch it. I grin to myself, knowing that I have reached it.

I played with that little spot inside of her a bit longer, listening to the change in her breath and feeling the fluids soaking my hand as I continued to lick her. Within seconds, I could feel her whole body spasm, and her vagina tightened and clenched on my fingers over and over again.

I pulled my hands away from her, knowing that she'll be far too sensitive for the next few moments to be of much fun. Instead, I turned to look over my shoulder at Matt. He was watching us intently as he thrust deeper. He had kept pace deep and slow while I tongued at Delilah, but now that I was done with her, he sped up, harder.

"Spank me," I managed to moan as he pushed deeper and deeper into me. I reached down between my legs to touch my clit, swollen and soaking wet, as he obliged, pulling out just long enough to slap both of my ass cheeks in quick succession. The sting felt so good, and just as quickly as he had stopped, he slammed himself into me again and again. I felt his hands tangle into my hair and pull my head back—it was uncharacteristically rough for him, and when I looked up at him, I could see his gaze fixated on me. He was completely in the moment, enjoying it.

"Play with her again," he said gruffly, shoving me down toward Delilah, who was watching us with heated passion.

I grinned, feeling wetter at the thought of my

husband, my usually so sweet and gentle husband, getting rough and hot and bothered by the idea of me fucking another woman. I could live with that. "My pleasure," I told him as he slowed down his fucking to let me keep my own balance.

I pulled Delilah closer to me, and she smiled up at me, her eyes begging for round two. I lined her up underneath me so that I could grind on her pelvis while I leaned down to kiss each of her perky little perfect nipples before taking one in my mouth.

I heard Matt's breathing pick up as he watched me, and I knew I needed to put on a show. Arching my back just right to bring my ass up for him, I leaned in to tug on Delilah's lips before I reached over to the nightstand next to our bed. I pulled out a toy—a large vibrator , which I quickly placed against Delilah's clit before settling my own right onto it as well, starting it on low. I gasped at the feeling, gliding my clit atop it as I watched Delilah's delicious expression on her face. It was perfect in that moment—she was so hot with her fuck-me eyes as she leaned up for a kiss, moaning against me. Matt's own tempo increased a bit, and I could feel his desperation as he fucked me harder. I heard him getting closer and closer and I pulled away from Delilah's mouth just long enough to look over my shoulder at him, making eye contact as he watched me. I turned away to suckle at Delilah's nipple again, but just as my lips grazed over the tiny little nub, he yanked my hair back.

"You'll look at me now," he practically growled, and I smirked at him. He thrust into me again, and my mouth opened, head back as he took me harder. I pushed harder against the vibrator that was underneath me, reaching down to turn up the speed.

Immediately, Delilah cried out in pleasure, and I pinched her nipples a little bit harder that time, never looking away from Matt as he continued to fuck me. Any time I started to close my eyes to enjoy the moment, he pulled my hair harder and forced me to keep my eyes on him. My pussy clenched his cock tighter as he forced me. Who knew I was into him being more dominant. It wouldn't be long—I knew I wouldn't be able to last out much longer as he continued to ride me.

"You don't cum until I tell you to cum," he told her, never letting up the intensity in his gaze or his fucking. All I could do was nod in response as another wave of pleasure threatened to throw me over the edge. The vibrator was too strong for me to be able to resist for too much longer, and I shifted off of it, leaving it in place for Delilah, who was practically in her own little world, enjoying herself. As soon as I was off of the vibrator, she took it with her free hand and plunged it into herself with a moan, her back arching, and eyes closing tightly.

Matt let go of my hair, and I looked down at Delilah, grinning at my handiwork, but before I could do much more, he thrust into me again, so hard that I could hardly stand it. I whined as he got deeper and deeper, and I knew he was challenging me. He *wanted* to make this hard for me, and could I really blame him? He was reclaiming his confidence—he *needed* to do this.

I tried to fend off the impending orgasm, but before I knew it, my vagina was tightening in waves of pleasure all down his shaft, and I felt him thrust harder into me and groan as well. I rode the waves of pleasure before collapsing onto Delilah, who smiled knowingly at me before she reached up to toy with my sensitive nipples.

She didn't get to for very long before I felt Matt's hand wrap around my arm, flipping me over. "You didn't listen," he told me, his eyes shining in dark amusement. I couldn't quite tell what he thought as he looked down at me.

"Sounds like I'm in need of a punishment," I replied coyly.

"Someone's a bad girl," purred Delilah with a giggle as she gently rubbed the vibrator along my clit. It was almost too sensitive to be enjoyable in the moment.

"Are you going to help me punish her?" asked Matt, looking at Delilah. "You'll get your reward when you're done."

This new side of Matt was so incredibly hot, and in that moment, I realized that this is exactly what we were missing in our own sex life. We were missing that carnal, intense, uninhibited pleasure that we were enjoying right that moment.

Delilah giggled sensuously as she lowered herself. "It's my turn to do the licking, I think," she murmured as she ran her tongue from my nipple all around my areola before lowering herself to lick at my stomach as well. She was so gentle, and her face was so smooth, in stark contrast to the looming form of Matt as he looked over his handiwork. My entire body was glistening with sweat, and my hair, once perfectly put in place, was tousled and knotting. He loved ravaging me and he loved looking at the ravaged body he left behind.

As Delilah slowly worked her way right back up to the other nipple, I moaned in pleasure. I could feel myself getting primed for another round already. My clit was twitching to attention, and my pussy ached to be filled again. I wanted this—I wanted to be dominated and controlled.

Matt watched as Delilah played with me. He watched the young woman's perfect figure move to straddle me, placing her clit against mine before rubbing. He watched as I gasped at the sudden shift and as my back begin to arch. His own cock was already hard and ready for round two, and he rubbed it slowly to keep his hands busy as Delilah's danced all over my skin. She was everywhere as she touched me; her hands never lingered too long in any place as she rode me, watching me. I felt myself getting wetter and more eager to continue playing the more that she rode me. I felt myself vying for her, and my own hips thrust upwards to meet her.

"No," Matt said.

I looked at him in surprise. No, what? He answered my silent question almost immediately.

"Don't move, or I'll have to tie you up."

I was shocked at what he said, but it only made me hotter. It only made me want to move to make him do it, but I found myself obeying. I didn't move as Delilah continued to ride me. I fought the urge to move, and she seemed to take it as a challenge to make me fail. She removed herself from me and lowered herself down to lick my slit, tasting the amalgamation of our juices that coated me as she did. Her tongue penetrated into me, and I gasped, but still managed to avoid moving. She licked me harder and harder, quickly taking the vibrator and turning it on as well, placing it against my clit. Her other free hand squeezed my ass, her nails digging into my skin just enough to pleasantly sting as she did so.

"Mmm..." I heard myself moan, and I looked at Matt in the eyes. He admired the work that was being done above me before lowering himself down. He took Delilah in front of him, positioned her just right, and thrust into her. The motion pushed her deeper into me and I could hear her gasp as he took her. I looked up and saw them fucking. He pulled her hair back, just as he had pulled mine, exposing a neck that he leaned down to nibble on before he sucked deeply onto it. I could hear the slurps as he sucked on her neck, marking her. I took a moment to catch my breath and reached down for the vibrator.

"Don't move," he repeated as he pulled Delilah back and fucked her harder. I obliged and sat there, watching him thrust his cock deeper into her, watching his balls bouncing and watching the ripples in his thighs as he held himself up and balanced them both. He was on his knees, as was she, her back arched so that he could reach her chest and her neck all at once. She moaned, eyes closed as she enjoyed the moment, and Matt maintained perfect eye contact with me as he took the vibrator that I had tried to use, turned it on, put it in place on Delilah, and finished the job.

Her head was thrown back in pleasure, mouth wide open and eyes squeezed shut. I could see her thighs tighten and contract as she came, and as soon as she was done, Matt let her go, shifting right back over to me without missing a beat or breaking eye contact.

"Don't move," he reaffirmed one last time as he watched me. "And you don't cum until I tell you to. Do you understand?"

"Yes," I breathed, watching him. My legs were quivering on their own, aching for his touch, and as soon as he spread my legs himself, I felt my breathing quicken almost immediately. I didn't move, and he thrust into me with abandon. He did not look away as he continued.

Before long, he yanked me up. "Turn around," he commanded, and I did so immediately. He pulled me into that same position to take me from behind, and got in deeply, pushing and thrusting as hard as he could into me. He pulled my hair and bit at my ear as he did so. I felt my breath gasping and felt his hands around my throat, not hard enough to completely cut off breathing, but just enough to put some pressure down as his cock reached deeper than ever before into me.

He grunted as he thrust, quicker and quicker, his shaft pulling out all but the tip of his head before thrusting it back in. "You're mine," he whispered into my ear gruffly as the pressure on my neck suddenly loosened. I had completely forgotten all about Delilah at this point, and quite frankly, I didn't care whether she was there or not. Matt shoved me down on the bed, slapping my ass with actual force behind it, so hard that I yelped, but that yelp of pain very quickly became a moan of pleasure as he buried his cock in me again, all the way to the balls. At this angle, they slapped against my clit just right, and he slammed into me, quicker and quicker.

"Cum for me now, or not at all," he told me suddenly, and he didn't have to say anything twice. As he buried his load in me, I felt myself clench all around him. I felt each thrust as he came before collapsing against me in a sweaty, exhausted heap. He pulled himself out of me and looked me over. My ass was red from the slaps, and my hair had gotten even worse. Delilah had apparently taken her leave while we were in the throes of abandon, but I was pretty sure she looked almost as disheveled as I did. I sighed, thoroughly fucked, thoroughly satisfied, and thoroughly ready for a nap.

"So, when's the next time?" Matt practically purred, running a hand up and down my arm, watching as I shivered in response. All I could do was laugh in response.

Clara's Experiment

Clara has never known what she wanted out of life. She was never very satisfied, and even though she always tried to enjoy herself, she decided that she wanted to try something new—she wanted to be dominated, and she wanted to do it with someone that she would never have to see again. Armed with the power of the internet, she finds someone to dominate her and goes for a night that she will never forget, meeting sexy, alluring Anthony in the penthouse suite of a hotel for a night of dark passion and submission that introduces her to a lifestyle she's not likely to forget anytime soon.

I looked down at my phone and saw an unbelievingly handsome face looking back at me. It was the profile for the man that I was heading to meet that evening, and I felt a pit of apprehension in my stomach. He looked like he was... Well, experienced, and it made me nervous. I had spent the night prior looking into doms online. It turns out; there are dating apps just like that. I'd never tried anything like that before, but a quick one-night stand seemed like an ample opportunity to get to know whether I'd like it or not.

The man's face was very serious. His skin was tanned, but not dark, and his gaze, intense. His profile picture showed that he meant business,

I noted—it was that of someone who knew what he wanted and was not willing to let anyone else prevent him from getting that, and that was exactly what I wanted. I was curious, vaguely, about the sub life, but had never had the guts, or the opportunity, to experiment with it myself. That was, until that night.

I stood at the bottom of a tall hotel, looking up at it, my phone still in hand. It was maybe 9:30 pm on a Friday night, and I was all dressed up. My makeup was expertly applied, and I wore red pumps with a short, form-fitting red dress that was stretched practically taut over my body. Underneath, I wore nothing—no bra, no panties, just as I had been told to do. I had to be careful when I leaned over or sit down or I'd run the risk of flashing someone, but that was a small price to pay for the pleasure I hoped to get that night. I was eager to give this a shot, that was for sure. I just had to get out and make it happen.

I took a deep breath. "Clara, get it together. You can do this!" I told myself, tightening my grasp around my phone before I stepped into the building with purpose. My head was held high and confident, despite feeling the exact opposite. I went up to the penthouse. I typed in a quick message into the dating app, informing him that I was on my way up, and I marveled at the fact that I would be setting foot into the area that would be deemed "high-class" or whatever else people say of the presidential suites in hotels. I had no idea what to expect as I made my way up the elevator to the room.

The elevator doors opened and revealed the man, Anthony, staring back at me. He was leaned against the wall, arms crossed casually, head back, and eyes glancing up and down as if trying to determine if I was worth the effort on that very night. He must have decided that I was, as he straightened up as soon as I stepped off the elevator. Did he think that I'd chicken out, maybe? Maybe he thought I'd just get right back on it and leave. Who knows? Whatever it was, though, I knew that I was in for a unique time. I had never seen anything like him before—his gaze was intense, but something in it was reassuring. I immediately felt at ease, something I had never experienced with a man before, certainly not a strange one that I had never met.

He looked at me and smirked. I was no longer standing tall—I was standing with my body relaxed as we walked. My arms were pulled in slightly... Almost submissively. He placed a hand on the small of my back, and I felt a thrilling jolt through me. I hadn't expected that at all, not that I could complain. It was nice.

Very quickly, we were inside the room, behind a closed door, and I stood, not really sure what to do next. I wasn't sure where I should be, and I looked around myself nervously. Thankfully, I didn't have to bring myself to ask. We hadn't yet exchanged a single word.

"Sit," he said. It wasn't a request—I could hear that. He wasn't yet looking at me, too busy rustling through a few things. I nodded my head to myself before moving to sit down on the bed. My head was spinning, but I obediently sat there without a care in the world. I was almost shocked at the fact that I was there without a protest, but I chose not to say a thing.

"Did you prepare yourself?" he asked. Anthony had given me several instructions—I was to be clean-shaven and without underwear when I arrived. Again, I nodded my head without a word.

He looked up to me briefly, almost questioningly. "I didn't hear you, Ellen."

Hearing my name on his lips brought a quick shiver down my spine. "Yes," I replied quietly. My voice quivered.

He stood up to full height as he looked over me, his dark eyes almost disapproving for a moment. "This is your first time," he said suddenly.

"Yes." I turned my gaze away from him.

He blinked, clearly taken aback by that. "You're... New and you were looking for partners on a dating app?" Something about the way that he said that made me feel a bit embarrassed. Had I made a mistake already? I had hoped to get everything just right.

"... Yes?"

He ran one hand through his hair, his gaze lifting off of me and focusing on something behind me as if considering something. "Look, had I known..." he began before I had to interrupt him.

"I want to learn."

"You need to learn some manners," he said with a smirk. I could see his hand tense at his hand, as if he had resisted the urge to smack me across my face. I shrank back slightly at the thought, but at the same time, I felt myself starting to get wet. I hadn't expected that, at all, but I was interested in seeing where things would go.

"I'm sorry," I told him contritely, looking at him.

"Look away," he commanded me, and I obeyed. "You have a lot of learning to do. Are you sure you want this?" In the corner of my eye, I could see that he was hard. He wanted to punish me. He wanted to discipline me and teach me what

I should and should not do. But, he also didn't want to get me in for more than I expected. After all, from everything I've read, this is about consent. Consensual abuse, basically. Or at least, that's how I understood it.

"I do want this," I told him, keeping my gaze planted firmly on his feet. It felt comfortable to look there, and I was looking at his brown shoes. They looked like leather, quite nice from what I could see.

"Okay," he replied simply after a pause. "Then let's begin. Safe words..."

With all of the niceties figured out, he grinned at me. It was a dark grin on his face, one that showed that he's more interested in using me than anything else. "Strip," he told me.

I nodded my head and grabbed the hem of my dress to pull it up. As soon as it was over my head, he swatted my now-bare ass swiftly with his hand, and I yelped at the sting. It started, but it was almost... pleasant? "What's that?" he practically purred, "I can't hear you."

"Yes, sir," I told him quietly, using the manners that he had just gone over with me.

"That's better."

He watched as I removed the dress, tossing it onto the bed. I was standing there, bare naked, aside from the red heels I had on. Red was his choice—he liked his gifts wrapped in red, he had told me. I looked at his feet a bit longer, watching as they walked in a circle to get a good look at his prize for the night. I got the feeling that I was being hung up for display, like a piece of meat, but somehow, the thought of being used like that only made me even more eager to please. He pushed me over the bed to take a look at me and pulled my lips and cheeks apart, viewing my pussy. He must have grinned—I couldn't see his reaction, but he gave each cheek a slap.

"Such a naughty little whore you are, aren't you," he practically purred, running a finger over my little nub, trailing down the outside of my lips and back again.

I gasped at the touch. I hadn't expected it so quickly, and yet, there it was. His fingers were gently, delicately, tantalizingly rubbing along my inner lips, careful to avoid the slit itself. He didn't want to move too quickly. I could feel myself begin to leak more, and he chuckled behind me. He was clearly fully satisfied, and he gave me another slap on both cheeks, harder this time. I yelped, and he let go. The sound of his footsteps said that he was leaving the area and I looked tentatively over my shoulder to see what he was doing.

Anthony had gone over to get something from a drawer, and I had to admit, I was a little afraid to see what he'd bring back. Quickly, I found that he had brought back a little riding crop. It smelled of leather as he put it down next to me. "You are to obey me and only me," Anthony said as he put down what looked like a strand of beads as well, and a toy that I couldn't quite tell what it was for. He grinned, but I hesitated to make eye contact with him.

"On your knees," he said suddenly, and I obliged. "Lean forward," he demanded.

I sat on the bed, on my knees, leaning forward so that my head rested against the bed. My ass was up in the air, and I felt the beads teasing at my pussy, a little at first. "Mmm," I purred as he let them go in, one at a time, inside of me. He let them all enter me and then quickly pulled them out. The feeling was shocking and unexpected and almost as good coming out as going in. I felt my pussy clench between my legs at the sudden absence of stimulation, but before I could protest, I felt him probing my asshole, gently at first.

"Have you ever had anything up here," he asked as he used what I assumed was his finger at first to poke at me. I was tight and clenching it in nervousness. I shook my head no, biting my lip and squeezing my eyes shut in anticipation for what I assumed was about to happen. "I don't hear you, slut," he said with a quick slap against my upper thigh.

"N-no, sir," I replied through clenched teeth. That had hurt, and yet, I felt myself grow wetter. I wanted this, I realized.

"Do you want it?" he asked me, and I saw him reach for the leather crop next to me.

"Yes, sir," I told him, and he snapped the crop against me. It stung, but just as quickly, he gently pulled it across the reddening skin, almost delicately, and I felt myself gasp. It moved slowly, moving to tenderly trace the outsides of my lips before gently tapping at those too. It was just enough to bring feeling there, barely brushing over them and I gasped at the sensation.

"Good," he growled, leaning over me to cup a breast that was hanging down on the bed. My nipples were brushing the sheets as he did it, and he reached up to bring them between his fingers, rolling them about until I moaned my pleasure. I loved it. I wanted it. I wanted more, and without saying a word, he obliged. He placed a couple of nipple clamps onto me, bringing a sudden gasp out of me. It was borderline painful, but another few traces around my lips and clit were enough to make me forget the pain in the moment.

He pulled my hair back, and I could see him watching me from the corner of my eyes. "Is this what you want, bitch?" he asked her, and I could see the steely amusement in his eyes. It was exactly the look I didn't know I wanted to see from him.

"Yes," I told him. He gripped my head harder. "Yes, sir!"

Anthony then took a moment to shove those beads, the beads that I had all but forgotten, into my ass, one at a time. Each bead that popped in made me gasp and shudder. Two... Three... Four... Five... My thighs were quivering, and I was barely holding myself up. The feeling was so foreign, but the weight within my ass was pleasant. I clenched around it.

"Good girl," he said with a slap, sending me gasping again. He flipped me over to look at his handiwork, and I laid there, palms up and at my head, turned to look at him from the side, and he grinned. "Good," he said, watching as my breath heaved in and out rapidly. My mouth was agape and I could feel the pressure within me building.

Without a word, he plunged his fingers inside of me, reaching up to find my g-spot, pressing against it. I shut my eyes and whined at the feeling, unable to help it as my thighs shot upwards in response, begging and pleading wordlessly for more than I had already gotten.

He chuckled darkly at me. "You think you're ready for this? For me?" he purred, leaning closer. He swatted at me with the crop just under my rib cage with a smirk. He was enjoying every moment.

"Y-yes, sir," I managed to just barely breathe out. I couldn't help it. I was spilling all over his bed; I could feel the wetness when he pushed me right down onto the mattress roughly. The sight only made him hotter, and I could see his dick hardening in his pants. He released it, revealing a solid seven inches—larger than average but not overwhelming. He rubbed it along my lips, his head tracing them, but never diving into the opening.

The feeling was enough to make me shudder and hitch my breath in my chest. My nipples were aching wonderfully under the weight of the clamps, and I reached toward his hips without thinking about it, preparing to pull him in.

Anthony pulled away, swiftly swatting both hands with his crop, leaving me crying out as pain met pleasure. "You do not touch me unless I tell you to," he told me curtly. "Do you understand, slut?"

"Yes, sir," I squeak out, rubbing my hands.

"Since you can't control your hands, I'll have to control them for you. Over your head, slut," he told me, and I obeyed as he walked around me, unwilling to give me the pleasure of feeling him against me by reaching over. He clenched both of my wrists and bound them together, putting them above me and into a bond to keep them from moving. The bond clipped to something on the headboard—I couldn't quite see it, but I could feel that it pulled my arms tightly. I tried to shift up to relieve some of the pressure.

"You stay here," he told me as he walked back to the other side of the bed and between my legs, pulling my hips back down toward him. I winced at the feeling of my wrists being pulled tightly but resisted making a sound. "Good girl."

As a reward for my obedience, he shoved his dick right into me, just as I had been waiting for. He pushed every inch in quickly, not giving me the chance to adjust to his length or his girth as he slammed against me. I caught my breath in my chest and whimpered as he did it again. His balls slammed into the beads in my ass, and I couldn't help but pull away a bit, only to meet his hands roughly holding me in place.

"You will stay here and take my cock like a good girl, do you understand me?"

"Y-yes."

"Good." He pushed in harder and harder, lifting the crop to tap it against each of the nipple clamps, evoking a scream from me as my hips slammed up to meet his as he thrust again. "Good, slut, take every inch of me."

"Give me every inch," I mewled in reply, breathing heavily. I was in heaven—I could feel the pressure of the beads within me rubbing pleasurably against the pressure of his cock as he continued to whip along me. It was so good... I was getting wetter within him, and I felt myself clench up around him.

"You are not to cum yet, do you understand?"

"Yes..." I breathed out between moans of pleasure. My head was back, eyes short, but I could hear him grunting as he sped up. He kept the rhythm, hard, fast, and deep, for a moment, his own breathing starting to hitch within him as well. He sounded so sexy in the moment as he used me like the toy that I knew I was meant to be. I wanted him to have me, and I let him pound me so hard that I thought I might tear under his pressure.

He groaned in pleasure as I felt his hips buck against me, leaving his load inside of me. He remained there, pushing against my hips for a few moments before he finally decided to pull away, looking at me like a piece of meat. He took a moment to catch his breath, his cock half-hard still, and shining in the dim light.

Wordlessly, he climbed up over me and dropped his balls in my face. "Lick them clean," he told me, and I obliged immediately.

I licked up every last drop of me from his balls and from his shaft, slowly and tenderly removing it. He was fully hard again by the time that I was done sucking on it and playing with it. "You have five minutes, suck me off, or you will be punished." Without a word, he set a timer and removed the restraints that had held me against the bed, though my hands were still together.

I obliged immediately, leaning down and taking as much of his girth as I could into my mouth. I lingered on the tip for a few moments, sucking it until I felt it twitch, and then I moved on to the shaft. Without my hands, I'd have to make do with just my mouth. I ran it into my throat as deeply as I could manage without choking and let my tongue squeeze against it, quickly pulling it out of my mouth and licking it from the balls up to the tip again and again.

The more that I sucked on him, the more I felt him twitching in my mouth and tried my best, but the timer came and went, and he flipped me over onto my back. He swatted me with the crop four times, hard this time, and I cried out at the feeling dancing. I was certain that the skin was welted at that point. "Nice try, but you failed," he told me as my eyes watered from the smarting welts underneath me.

"I'm sorry, sir," I told him, wincing. All I wanted at that point was to finish. I was going insane, feeling the weight of the beads within me, and I was getting desperate.

"Your punishment," he told me, "is that you will be fucked without being allowed to cum, do you understand me?"

"Yes, sir," I said back, despite feeling like I wanted to protest. It was almost like my body and mind wanted two different things. He slammed his cock into me again, once again hard, and he worked me up, slamming in harder and harder. He could feel me getting close and pulled out just before I was able to cum, leaving me collapsing against the bed, frustrated.

"What's wrong?" he asked, leaning over me with that same smirk on his face. "Frustrated?"
"No, sir."

"Oh, I see," he said, prying my legs apart. He lowered his head to lick at my clit, his tongue dancing gently around the protected little nub. He licked up and down it slowly, sensually, watching as my body tensed up in response. He lowered his tongue to dance on the outside of my lips, teasing the entrance just barely with a flick of his tongue before bringing it right back up to the top again. He sucked on the little nub, his tongue dancing on and around it as he did.

His finger snaked up to penetrate me, slowly pushing into me as he did. He looked up at me from his place, eating at me and watched as my back arched and I moaned loudly in pleasure. I couldn't take it... I felt the pressure building up, and I didn't think that I could hold it back anymore...

And he pulled away. He looked at me from his position and stood up over me.

"The little slut doesn't deserve to finish tonight after failing me," he told me with a quick swat of the crop against my skin, leaving me wanting desperately without anything to relieve myself. I groaned as I fell down onto the bed, and he smirked again.

"Then again... You are a new little slut, aren't you? Do you want to beg for release?"

"Please," I said suddenly, my voice pleading. My pussy was dripping and empty, and I wanted something—anything—in it.

"Please, what?"

"P-please fuck me," I cried out in desperation.

"What's that?"

"Sir, please, fuck me sir!" I moaned, fighting the urge to reach for him. My body couldn't take the buildup any longer, and before I could say another word, he pushed himself into me again. I gasped, shuddering at the feeling. It was exactly what I needed, and I writhed on the bed, thrusting my body against his.

"Cum for me, slut," he commanded firmly.

I felt my body oblige immediately. I felt the clench of pressure in my pussy as it gripped against his dick. I felt the waves of release that I had been waiting for all evening, giving way around him, over and over, for what felt like forever as he finished within me. I felt his release alongside mine, and he pulled himself out of me.

My breathing was heavy, and I was exhausted beyond belief, eyes still closed. My whole body ached pleasantly under the strain and release. I felt the nipple clamps release off of me, and I looked up to see Anthony watching me. He smirked self-satisfied. "Now, get out of my sight, you slut. I'll see you tomorrow."

He didn't even have the courtesy to ask—just assumed that I'd be back again. He wasn't wrong.

Amelia's Punishment

Amelia is a housekeeper that has a strange job. Every week, she's asked to come over and clean, wearing a skimpy outfit for a man that rarely ever says more than a word or two to her at a time. She cleans the spotless surfaces for the money but finds herself getting paid more than she ever thought she could ask for when she accidentally drops a crystal glass and needs to be punished for her transgressions by her sexy boss, Mr. Erikson, who wants nothing more than to rip her skimpy little outfit off of her and ravish her body.

Even though the area was always immaculately clean, I was still always asked to come over every week to dust, wipe, and polish anything that I found on the shelves. It was mildly humiliating; Mr. Erikson required me to wear this skimpy little maid's outfit that barely covered my ass cheeks, but let's be real here for a moment—I *loved* having my cheeks hang out. Sometimes, if Mr. Erikson, the fine specimen of a man that he was, was looking my direction, I'd intentionally stand up on my tippy toes to reach out to some imagined hard to reach area *just* to give him a flash of my ass. No panties. That part was all me, not him. I imagine that he'd get hard at his desk, hidden behind the wooden surface, as I reached up. I imagined that he'd let his eyes slowly take me in as stretched. I imagined that he was an ass man, based on the fact that mine was just barely covered, but to be fair, my dress barely covered my tits either—it pushed them up, almost uncomfortably tight, to create a huge cleave down my front as they were smashed together. I looked good, that was for sure, and I always had to wonder if he only wanted me here so that he could have some eye candy. After all, there were rarely any real messes for me.

I was busy scrubbing some invisible splotch on the wall, over and over, slowly just rubbing my towel on the wall. Sometimes, I'd sit there and sensually begin to clean objects, suggestively running my fingers up and down the length of an ornate crystal decanter filled with amber liquid. It was rum, maybe, or brandy or whiskey. I never opened it up, but I did know that the amount of liquid in the bottle was always changing from week to week when I did my rounds, so it must have been for more than just decoration.

That day, I could feel Mr. Erikson watch me with mild disinterest as if I weren't there. His gaze would drift over to me, and I'd feel tension in the air, but he must have been distracted. It was like he saw right through me as his eyes caressed my legs, lazily going up and down their lengths, but his mind was clearly elsewhere. I'd have to try harder if I wanted him to actually look at me. The idea of a challenge made my pussy twinge in anticipation. We never fucked or anything. In fact, we never even touched or said more than just a few terse words to each other, but the tension in the air was palatable. I bet Mr. Erikson could have cut the tension with his dick. I knew he liked watching me; the bulge that he had in his pants the few times he walked by, unabashedly unconcealed, told me that much.

I'd have to try harder; I told myself if I wanted to win that day. I wanted that sexual tension to build up so much that I could hardly take it. I'd never actually initiate; the job paid too well to just be eye candy. But, I'd be lying if I said that I didn't regularly think about throwing myself on the desk and begging him to take me on more than one occasion.

As I worked on cleaning up the wall, then, I let the rag slip out of my hand to the floor. Honest mistake, right? I bent down, keeping my knees straight, revealing myself to Mr. Erikson. Considering the clattering of his pen that I heard, he must have seen it all, and I smirked, feeling another twitch in my pussy. My clit was starting to swell, and I could feel the fluids beginning to soak everything. Slowly, I straightened up without a word, discarding the rag and getting a clean one, and I moved on to polishing the glasses that matched the decanter. They were smooth and felt hefty in my hand, the cool crystalline surface shining brilliantly in the light of the office. The office was kept dark most of the time, curtains drawn and warm lamps on creating just enough light for Mr. Erikson to do whatever it was that he did at his desk. I wasn't sure what he did—I had never thought to ask him, nor did I really care. We didn't talk much. My job was to clean everything and I was not allowed to leave for the whole two hours that I was paid to be there to clean it. At first, the two hours seemed to drag on forever, but our unspoken game made the time fly by when I wasn't paying attention to it. I gently placed the glass back down and picked up the next one, polishing that one as well. I would imagine that they were his cock, hard and smooth in my hand, as the towel rubbed up and down, polishing even the bottom of it. My fingers would linger, rubbing sensually on the crystal surface. I'd do them one by one before putting them perfectly down where they had been before. As I reached to put the last glass down, it slipped from my hand and clattered as it fell onto the ground, thankfully onto a rug. I froze when I realized what happened.

"Amelia?" I heard him speak—he never spoke if he could avoid it.

"Yes, sir?" I managed to force myself to say, my voice shaking. I was shocked that I had made such a mistake—I was usually so careful with what I did. It was highly abnormal for me to make mistakes like that. Everything was calculated and planned out, but I had gotten careless.

I heard Mr. Erikson's chair move out from behind his desk, and I could hear the rustling of his clothing as he stood up. He was looking right at me, but I couldn't bring myself to even look at him. I had done it now! I knew I'd be fired on the spot—I'd heard rumors in the house that he was always firing the house staff if they didn't exceed his expectations! I groaned inwardly.

"Amelia." He was firmer this time as my name escaped his lips, sending a shiver down my spine. Despite the concern for being fired, I *still* wanted him. Hell—half of me hoped he'd bend me over the desk and spank me for my punishment and let me get back to work.

I forced my eyes to slowly shift over to him; my gaze slowly drifting across his body from the ground up. When I made it to his cock, my eyes widened, seeing it swollen and bulging against his pants, threatening to destroy the zipper if it wasn't freed soon. His pants were black, crisply ironed and somehow, without a single wrinkle in them, despite working at a desk. He was toned—or at least, I assumed he was toned by the shape of his arms when he'd work, bulging and rippling. He clearly exercised regularly. When I finally raised my gaze to meet his own icy cool one, I was greeted with the sight of a barely perceptible smirk. If I didn't know him better, and to be frank, I barely knew him at all; I'd say that he was giving me bedroom eyes— you know the kind that says that you're ready to throw the person onto the bed and fuck their brains out kind of eyes.

And it made me so hot.

"You've been a naughty girl, Amelia," he said, his voice quiet and in control as he looked me over. I was shrinking into myself, making myself as small as possible. My arms were crossed in front of me, pushing my breasts up further in their skimpy little covering that could hardly be considered covered in the first place.

"I'm sorry sir," I managed to squeak out in response.

And he chuckled. It was a dark chuckle, sensuous as he looked me over like he was considering something. "You better be." Something about the veiled threat sent a thrill running down my spine. "Do you know what we do to naughty girls around here, Amelia?"

"N-no sir." I had some high hopes, though.

"They are punished according to their crimes. Do you know why that glass is always here?"

"No..."

"No, what?"

"No, sir."

"Good girl." He smirked, one brow raising up as he did. He was checking me out. "That was my late father's set. It is irreplaceable."

I hadn't realized, and suddenly, I felt bad. It wasn't broken; somehow, it had managed to land on a rug and didn't break, thankfully, but I still felt *awful*. "What is my punishment, sir?" My gaze was firmly on his feet at this point. I couldn't explain it, but all of my confidence that I had had just moments prior had all melted away.

"You need a spanking, Amelia." I heard him cracking his knuckles then, and I looked up at him in surprise. His dick was harder than ever, judging by the fact that his pants had somehow become even tauter than they had been just moments prior, and I looked at him in awe. Was he going to fuck me? I kind of hoped he did. My fear melted away as he beckoned for me to move closer to him, and I did it without a single protest.

Suddenly, I felt his hands wrap around my wrist and pull me close. I could smell his aftershave; he smelled clean and strong with a hint of subtle spiciness, and I loved it. His fingers on my skin were strong and warm, firm, but not painful, and he placed his other hand on the small of my back, wordlessly telling me to bend over, and I did, my body resting atop his desk. He was strong and firm; I couldn't

64

help but want to obey, even as I felt the first
sting of his strong, warm hand hitting my bare
ass. I squealed in surprise, bucking back at the
sudden surprise of the movement, sending a
pen holder clattering to the ground. I tried to
pull away, but he firmly pressed into the small
of my back. He wanted me to stay there.

"You've been such a naughty girl," he
practically purred in my ear, his voice low and
husky. I could hear the desperation in it. He
wanted this just as much as I did. I didn't
protest as I felt his hand slowly rubbing over
my ass, giving it a firm squeeze as he did. Then
both hands groped at me, pulling my cheeks
apart. "You have such a tight little ass," he
marveled under his breath. "I'm going to make
it mine."

I gasped as he pressed his cock against me. It
was hard and larger than I had thought in his
pants. He leaned over me, letting his hands
slide up my whole body from my ass, up my
back, and sliding around my waist and up
higher to grasp my tits, squeezing them tightly.
He fondled them, letting his hand squeeze a bit
tighter than I had expected. With the weight of
him atop me, I felt my heart pounding in my
chest, and I gasped. I fought the urge to turn
my head to kiss him. I was so wet at that point.
I'm sure it was soaking through his pants as he
continued to grind his cock against me. I could
feel myself practically dripping between my
thighs as he kneaded at my nipples, slipping his

fingers into the tight top of the dress. He didn't even bother fighting with it; he just tore it off, literally tearing down the front, and I didn't say a word. It was almost hotter to see the display of strength as he did it.

With my breasts free, he pulled at them before pulling back. Then, unexpectedly, I felt another slap against my ass. It was strong, and it was painful, almost immediately. I cried out at the sudden impact, but it was more in shock than anything else.

"What a naughty, dirty little slut you are," he breathed in my ear as he leaned over me again. "You're dripping." His breath on my neck sent shivers down my spine, and I turned my head just slightly, granting him access to do whatever he wanted to it, and he obliged. His lips fell on my neck and I felt his tongue dance across my skin before he nipped and nibbled. He wasn't rough enough to hurt, but I was sure I'd need to wear a scarf for the next few days.

He pulled back, and again, I felt another slap on my ass, but this time, he didn't pull his hand away. He let his hand linger against my skin. "Do you like your punishment?" His fingers slid closer to my slit, close enough to feel my wetness all over them.

"Yes, sir," I breathed out, tensing up and pushing my ass out just enough to try to encourage him to enter me. He pulled his fingers away from me, teasing the lips with the lightest of touches. He wasn't going to let me enjoy things that easily.

"Good. I don't tolerate little dirty sluts that don't know their place. You're going to learn your lesson tonight, do you hear me?"

"Yes, sir." I felt him let go of my ass and slap me again, and I cried out at the strange immersion of pain and pleasure as he did it.

Mr. Erikson flipped me over onto his desk and lifted me up as if I weighed nothing, setting me down atop it to get a full view of his handiwork. He looked at my breasts, no longer covered up by the black fabric that was in tatters around my waist, as if considering something, and then tore it all the way off. "You don't need this, do you?"

I shook my head breathlessly, in awe at the strength of the man in front of me. He leaned over me, his hands resting on either side of my legs, his nose so close that I could have touched it just by leaning forward. The urge to kiss him grew harder, and I leaned in to do it, only to feel his hand pulling my hair back to stop me. I squealed and looked up at him.

"You do not touch me. I touch you. You are here for me."

"Yes, sir," I said, trying not to struggle against the tugging on my hair.

He released my hair and pushed me down onto the desk, unzipping his pants and releasing the largest cock I had ever seen. No wonder his pants looked so tense against the heft of it. He pushed it against me, and I could feel it, hot and pulsating against my thigh. He rubbed it on me, up and down, and I could feel it gliding over me. The rubbing on me seemed to turn him on more, and he suddenly rammed it straight inside of me without hesitation.

I felt his big cock fill me up until I felt like I couldn't possibly expand any further, and yet, he kept pushing it in, forcing it deeper until I wondered if I would split in half. He held it there, tense and deep within me, and I realized he still hadn't gone all the way.

"Your wet pussy is so tight," he growled in my ear. He gyrated his hips just enough to press against my inner walls, and I moaned in pleasure. It was a tight fit, but that made it even better. I clenched against him as he slowly pulled himself out, and he thrust in again and again. "I will ravish this pussy tonight, do you hear me?"

I could barely manage to speak at the feeling of his cock rubbing against me. It was like a dream come true—I had fantasized about this moment so much, and here it was, happening.

"Amelia. Do. You. Hear. Me." He thrust in deeply between each and every word he said, making me moan every single time. I was breathing heavily, looking up at him, my mouth agape. I could hardly control myself enough to speak.

"Y-yes, sir," I managed to breathe between thrusts. His cock was better than I could have possibly imagined.

"Do you want me to take this pussy?"

"Yes!" I cried out, throwing my head back, bracing myself against the desk. He reached out and grabbed my breasts, weighing them in his hands. He was rough, but not hurtful as he ran his thumbs over my nipples, tracing circles right around them with the pads of his thumbs resting right onto them. My eyes were shut, enjoying the sensations of my body as he continued to thrust within me. I could feel the tension building up in pleasurable waves as he occasionally flicked and twisted at my nipples between thrusts.

I could feel myself getting close, and my breathing hitched in my chest as he continued to thrust inside of me. He would go faster and slower. Sometimes, he would almost tenderly and slowly pull it out and push it back in, other times, he would thrust his cock into me so rapidly that he had to hold me in place so I wouldn't fall off of the desk.

More items clamored to the floor, landing near the torn and discarded maid's costume. Just when I thought I wouldn't be able to take it any longer, he pulled out of me, looking at me in dark amusement. He was enjoying taking charge. "You're not cumming 'til I tell you that you can," he informed me as he flipped me over and pushed me back. I was standing on the floor now, on my tiptoes, and my arms and torso were stretched out across the surface of the desk. He spanked me again, hitting atop an area that had already been swatted earlier, and it stung enough to make me hiss in pain, but before I could protest, his cock was right back inside of me, making me forget all about the stinging.

He stayed there for just a moment or two, and as soon as I could feel myself getting close again, he stopped. "You're such a dirty little wench, aren't you, getting close already? Control yourself." He took my hand this time and led me to a door in the back of his office that I had never entered before. As soon as he opened the door, he revealed that there was a large, walk-in closet, but it was entirely devoid of any hangers or jackets, or even office supplies. Instead, there was a large, thick pole that went from wall to wall, and there were restraints suspended for it, thick and black and appearing strong enough to hold someone up. I hesitated, looking at it, but felt Mr. Erikson's cock against my back, wet and chilled by the ambient air. It pressed against me firmly, ushering me to enter, and I did, slowly turning around to look at him. Now we were in uncharted territory for me, but I wasn't sure that I really cared. I wanted this man's cock in me as hard as it could be to get me off as soon as possible and he seemed to sense that based on the fervor with which he wrapped his fingers around my delicate wrists and tied me up. It wasn't so bad; I told myself as I felt the restraints. They were tight against my wrist, but they didn't hurt. They held my hands right above my head and kept me from being able to move them too much, but it was okay with me. I didn't mind—until suddenly, he tightened the restraints and I felt my arms being yanked upward. I had to stand on my toes to keep the pressure from getting to be too much for me.

Mr. Erikson looked over my body carefully, eyeing my tits and my hips and the dip between them. He spread my lips between my legs and smirked as he did. "You've quite the body here. Why have you teased me so much with it?" His gaze flitted to mine for a fleeting instant, and I saw that intense desire burning within them. I smirked back, but just as quickly as I did, I felt a quick stinging across my thighs as he slapped them. I could see the handprints welting immediately.

"Did you want me?" he asked me after a moment.

"I did, sir," I replied, licking my lips slowly. I could see him watching me do it. I wanted him to want me right that moment so that we could fuck more. I stood up taller, thrusting out my chest, hoping that he'd give in and take me right then and there.

He ran his fingers up and down my thighs before slipping them between my legs, reaching up to touch that tiny nub folded away in my lips. He touched my clit, and I felt my legs immediately begin to quiver. I moaned softly at the contact, my hips thrusting. I felt his fingers trail further downward, and he traced my slit, pushing against it, but never actually penetrating me. His fingers slid further back than that, too—his fingers danced around my asshole, pressing on it. His finger, still wet with my juices, penetrated just slightly, slowly making its way into me. "Have you ever been fucked here before?"

"N-no sir," I gasped out as he pushed his finger deeper into me. I felt my muscles contract around his finger, and he put a second finger in as well, moving it in and out. After a few moments, he added in a third as well, gently penetrating just enough to get the muscles used to it. I felt myself starting to relax as he continued, and the sensation excited me further. The feelings of pleasure bloomed, and I

found myself loving it, and then his fingers
pulled out altogether.
I felt a dildo, larger than his fingers, thrust into
my slit, pushing and twisting it deeper and
deeper, and I felt the pleasure begin to build up
even more. My pussy was swelling with
anticipation as the sensations grew stronger,
and he pulled the toy out, immediately pressing
it against my ass again before slowly easing the
toy in. "We'll have to work up to my cock. I
wouldn't want to tear you in half," he said with
a smirk as he slid the toy into me. I was on my
tiptoes still, desperately trying to keep my legs
from giving out underneath me as the pleasure
threatened to overcome me, and just as quickly
as it had started, he pulled it out and removed
the restraints. I practically collapsed under the
weight of myself, but he caught me and lowered
me to the ground, positioning me on my hands
and knees with my ass in the air. He pumped
his cock into me a few times, lubricating
himself with my own fluids, of which there was
no shortage, before easing himself into my ass.
His cock was massive, and I didn't think that it
would fit, but still, it plunged deeper and
deeper. I threw my hand backward with a
moan of pleasure, and he wrapped his hand
around me, reaching for my throat. He put
pressure on it as he fucked me harder, not
enough to cut off my windpipe, but just enough
to elevate the sensation as he continued. He
thrust harder and harder into my ass, and I
could feel him getting harder inside my tight
ass until finally, he groaned in pleasure,

thrusting deeply and holding me there as he released his cum into me before pulling out slowly.

"Hold that cum in you. Don't let a drop fall out," he told me as he stood up, straightening out his tie and fixing his pants. I stayed on my hands and knees as he cleaned himself up, clenching my ass and feeling endlessly frustrated. He flipped me over. "Now, I can see that the dirty slut didn't finish with my cock, is that so?"

"Yes, sir," I told him, feeling the ache growing more than before. I wanted to fuck still, but he had other plans. He smirked at me. "Make your dirty pussy cum for me, but don't lose a drop of what I left in you," he commanded, crossing his arms and leaning back. I was taken aback by the command, but it wasn't the worst thing in the world. It would be the perfect way to entice him back for another round later. After all, I worked there several times a month.

I reached around, still on my hands and knees, using one hand to gently touch myself. I felt just how wet I was; I was practically dripping. My ass was still up in the air, and Mr. Erikson got the full view of my fingers, gently caressing my lips and rubbing on my clit as I did. I ran my fingers over the opening slowly at first, then pressed them in, one at a time, moaning sensually as they penetrated me. I reached in deeper, angling my fingers upward, touching at my g-spot within me, and I felt my hips thrust themselves in pleasure. I ran my fingers in deeper and deeper into myself, feeling every clench of my inner walls, every time I tightened and every shudder, and finally, within moments, I felt the pleasure welling up within me. I could feel the climax peaking, threatening to erupt, until it finally exploded, sending my hips and my vagina into spasms around my fingers, tensing up tighter and tighter, over and over again.

As the pleasure subsided, leaving my body pleasantly buzzing, I slowly pulled my fingers out from within me and looked at Mr. Erikson, who was watching with great interest, and I slowly licked my fluids off of myself. I sucked them clean, never breaking eye contact with him, even when I could see his pants start to tighten around his crotch again. "I can't wait for you to punish me again. I might have to even do some naughty things on purpose next time," I practically purred as I stood up to look at him.

He smirked back at me. "I'll just have to punish you harder next time."

Unwrapped Gifts

Nora loves her boyfriend and wants to give him a present for his birthday that he'll never forget, so she wraps herself up with her best friend for as long as she can remember, Becca, and sets herself up for some steamy action for Jared, happy to give him a day that he'll remember for years to come. Together, the naughty women enjoy themselves a little too much and leave him aching for more and looking for as much of a fuck as he can get. The lucky guy gets to unwrap two presents at once and enjoy every moment of it.

It was Jared's birthday, and I had a big plan in store for him. It was going to be the greatest birthday of his life, and he had no idea yet. I grinned at my friend, Becca, who was next to me. She was drop-dead gorgeous. She had naturally auburn hair that fell in waves and the greenest eyes that I had ever seen, and her lightly tanned skin was dusted with freckles right atop her perfectly sculpted cheekbones that sat high. She was wearing sultry makeup that day, her eyes shadowy and perfectly done, and she had a skintight, short dress with a deep v plunge, showing off the perfect cleavage she had.

Becca was my best friend and had been for years. She was someone that I was willing to share just about anything with—and I mean *anything*. As we smirked at each other, we knew that we were in for quite the night. I reached out to touch her arm, and she looked at me for a moment. "Are you sure about this, Nora?"

"Of course! It can't be too bad, can it? Besides, don't you remember our experimental phase in college?" It was true—we had been quite willing to explore each other's bodies and the wonders that they brought with each other when we were roommates, especially after a few nights of too many drinks.

She smiled widely, her eyes sparkling. She knew I had a point, but it wasn't every day that you fuck your best friend with your boyfriend. She put a hand on my back gently, and I hugged her. We would have a good time, that much I was sure of. I just had to be willing to actually do it, and I was sure that, in the moment, the look on Jared's face when he realizes that his birthday gift is literally his dream, being able to fuck two women at once, he would love every moment of it.

"What do you say we pre-game a bit?" asked Becca, looking at me through her lashes, her lips tugging upwards just slightly. She raised one brow as she did, waiting for my response. That didn't sound like that bad of an idea, I told myself. Besides, watching me get it on with a girl was another one of his biggest fantasies, and he was due to be home any time now.

I leaned in toward Becca, planting a kiss on her lips gently, and as I pulled back, she dove in for more. She pulled me in greedily, savoring the taste of my lips as she bit onto them, her tongue skating across them as she sucked. Her eyes were closed as she enjoyed herself, moaning against my lips. Her hand snaked around my neck, wrapping itself into my hair to hold me in place tightly in her passion. We weren't in love or anything, but who said a couple of girls couldn't platonically enjoy their body together in peace?

I reached up toward her breasts, feeling them gently with my palms. Her nipples hardened underneath the weight of my hand, pressing against my skin, and I could tell that she liked it by the way she kissed harder. Her hands twisted in my hair and one of her hands dropped down to rub on the outside of my own dress, right on my crotch area. We were careful not to mess each other up too much—we were all dressed up for Jared to unwrap. But, we could still tease each other and that we were doing.

Becca's breasts were so soft under my hand. Seriously, women's tits were like nature's greatest stress balls. The more I played with her, and the more she rubbed up against me, the less nervous I became. I found myself stroking her thighs, up and down, letting my fingers skate across the smooth, perfectly waxed surface. I was on her inner thigh, feeling the softness and the warmth emanating from just above. I could smell her moistness, soft, sweet, feminine, and carnal all at once, and it just made me want to play with her more. I let my fingers sneak their way up her dress to rub against the thin fabric of her panties. They were lace, and they weren't doing much at all to contain the juices that were beginning to flow. They were damp already, and I was able to slip my finger around them to touch the waxed pussy that was waiting for me. She was so warm and so soft under my fingers, and as soon as I let them graze over the lips between her legs, I felt Becca's kissing grow more desperate. Her pelvis tensed and her hips thrust forward, and I felt her legs spread apart just enough to let my had have more access. I reached up to touch her clit, rubbing it gently and tracing circles around it. I could feel it twitching and throbbing under my finger, telling a tale of how much she was enjoying the moment. Her breath caught in her chest and suddenly, she was practically silent and still, feeling my touch.

I reached my other hand to knead at her breast, rubbing it in between my fingers as I did. She loved every moment of it, and she couldn't hide it, even if she wanted to. I smiled as I slammed into her lips again, letting my tongue slip between her lips to taste hers this time. My fingers rubbed up against her over and over again before finally slipping inside of her. Her pussy was so tight against my fingers as I pushed in, feeling her inner walls clench against me. She wanted me to push into her, and I did, over and over again. I pushed harder and harder until I could feel her practically writhing underneath the weight of my hand.

She was so tight with my fingers in her, and I plunged deeper, twisting my fingers within her. I could feel her body begin to tense up more and more until I made her cum with a loud moan, head thrown back and hair draped down, exposing her long, slender neck as the waves of pleasure shook her body.

I kissed against her neck as I waited for the waves to subside, and when they did, she looked at me lustily, grinning. Her hair was mussed, but it just made her look hotter. She leaned over me, pinning me to the wall, ready to return the favor as she pushed her fingers around the tiny black thong I was wearing and stroking my clit. The sensation zapped throughout me, earning a throaty moan, and she pressed harder. She was touching me harder, tugging at my hair with her other hand so that she could wrap her lips around my neck and suck on the skin.

Her fingers expertly stroked over my clit as it swelled and pulsed until a finger slid into me. She curled her fingers up, and I felt myself tightening up as she stroked the inside of my pussy walls. I felt myself gyrate my hips, pushing her hand deeper. "You feel so good," I whispered to her between deep breaths as she teased me more and more. I wanted her deeper as I pushed against her hand, and she obliged, reaching her other hand to grope at my breasts instead, teasing my nipple underneath her fingers. I was practically whimpering at that point as she continued to fuck me with her fingers. Her mouth nibbled and licked at my neck and my ears as her fingers continued to knead me through the cloth. My body was shaking underneath the weight of her body and before I knew it, I was cumming around her fingers, feeling the pleasure overcome me for what felt like forever.

When I finally regained my senses, I opened my eyes to look at Becca, only to see Jared with an awestruck face right behind her. He had dark hair and skin, and his eyes were nearly black, but in the moment, he was slack-jawed, and I could see the erection growing in his pants. Who knew how long he had been watching, but he had certainly liked what he had seen enough to let us continue, completely uninterrupted.

Becca, seeing my focus shifted somewhere else, turned around to see what had caught my attention and smiled her sexiest smile, leaning forward and putting her hands in front of herself, clasped together so that her breasts were squeezed and pushed up. "Happy birthday, birthday boy!" she purred as she leaned over to run a hand up and down his chest, just as we had planned.

"We've got a great day in store for you," I chimed in, leaning over and planting a kiss right on his face, letting my hands slide down to rub against his hard cock in his pants. I unbuttoned him right there. "I'll unwrap you first so you can unwrap your gift." His pants were quickly discarded, as was his shirt, leaving him there, naked and wonderfully toned, not unlike a Greek statue—the ones where every single bulge is in the right spot. But this statue had one extra part—a long, rock-hard cock that was ready for action. I touched it, feeling it twitch underneath the touch.

He looked at me and then at Becca, and it finally seemed to register. "Really, babe?" he asked, and I nodded in response with a sly smile. I was glad that he seemed eager to enjoy his gift, and I took him by the hand and led him to our bedroom. We had a king bed so there was plenty of room for anything that we wanted to do. We could both lay together there no problem, even with Becca. We weren't exactly big women by any means; we were both maybe 5' even and petite, in perfect contrast to Jared's 6' and muscular build.

As we got into bed, I felt Jared's hand slap my ass, and I squealed and giggled in response. We were definitely in for a fun time. "What do you want us to do?" I asked him in my sweetest voice. "We'll do *anything*." I really emphasized that last word, letting it hang with a suggestive waggle of my eyebrows that got him to chuckle to himself.

"Anything?"

"Anything," we both replied, hoping that he wouldn't come up with some off-the-wall answer about what it was that he actually did want. We waited for him quietly, looking at each other.

"Striptease," came his reply after what felt like forever.

We grinned. We could do that. And so, we did. I reached over to Becca, letting my hand rub along her neck as I grasped the lining of her dress before pulling it over her head, revealing her naked body for Jared to see. I looked at her—she had gone braless, which explained exactly why I had been able to feel her nipples so easily, and I tossed her shirt aside, looking at the beautiful, pink circles in the center of her breasts. I wanted to suck on them, and I leaned in to plant the lightest of kisses on each nipple, watching them stand to attention after doing so before letting Becca do the same to me. My dress was also discarded, but my thong and bra were left on.

"Remove her panties with your teeth," Jared told me suddenly, and I'm not going to lie—that caught me off guard. But, I did it anyway, leaning in closely to Becca's leg and sensually rubbing along the skin before reaching up with my mouth to wrap myself around the lace. I could smell her arousal; she was dripping even more now than she was before as I pulled the panties down carefully with my teeth, getting a glimpse of her perfect bare ass. Seriously, Becca was a goddess of a woman.

"Play with each other some more," commanded Jared, and we both obliged immediately. After all, he *was* the birthday boy—what he wanted, he would get. We just had to be willing participants for his every whim. Becca took charge first, leaning over me on the bed. Her perfect, perky tits hung over my face, tantalizingly teasing with every movement she made. I reached up to caress her nipples, and she leaned down to remove my bra, tossing it to the floor with abandon. She leaned down, looking up at Jared and holding his gaze as she kissed each of my nipples and let her tongue snake out of her mouth, licking the areolas, careful not to ever touch the nipple itself. She teased around the nipple, leaving it erect and longing. It felt good, but I found myself desperate for her touch, my own arousal

84

growing with each and every lazy circle around the top of my breast. She moved to the other, slowly circling around the nipple again, leaving me breathless. She let her breath linger over it, watching as Jared stroked himself to us.

He loved his private show, his cock hard and long in his hand as he slowly, almost lazily, went up and down its shaft. I watched him touch himself and felt myself get wetter at the thrill of knowing that we were driving him crazy with every movement we made.

Becca slid down, kissing my taut stomach as she made her way down to my crotch little by little, she kissed the mound at the top. She let her tongue taste me, but only tracing the outer lips of my labia, driving me insane. I felt my hips thrusting of their own accord, silently betting her to touch, and I could feel the wetness beginning to accumulate, and then be licked up greedily by Becca's swift tongue.

She teased me up more and more, knowing that she was driving me crazy. I always loved being licked up and down, and she knew that more than anyone else—but I still was denied.

And just as quickly as it began, it stopped as Jared came over to get between us. His cock was hard in his hand, and I could see the desire in his eyes as he looked at both of us, almost as if choosing which one of us he wanted to get to fuck first. His eyes rested on me as if waiting for my approval, and when I nodded my head, he turned to Becca and grabbed her shoulder, spinning her around. Her eyes widened for a moment, but she didn't protest as he pushed her to the bed.

He rubbed his cock on her clit, and I could see her pleasure clear as day as she moaned, head back before he pushed deep into her with a hard thrust. He was quick with his thrusts, going as deep as possible. His balls slapped against her ass over and over, and he let out a groan of pleasure as he reached forward to greedily paw at her breasts, holding them in his hand and squeezing.

Just as quickly as he started fucking her, he reached over to grab me and pull me over next to her. He pushed his hands inside of me as well, letting his rough fingers penetrate deeply and stroke my inner walls as he tried to please me as well. He had one hand on Becca's breast, his cock deep in her, and his other hand inside of me as I reached down to touch my clit as well, with another hand on my breast, tugging at my nipples.

He fucked harder and harder into Becca until her moans of pleasure became cries of utter ecstasy, so loud that if we had been in an apartment, I would have worried about neighbors hearing us. He fucked deeper and deeper into her, focusing on the sensation, his fingers slipping out from me and shoved into her face, which she happily lapped up, taking my taste into her mouth and sucking on them. He groaned again with one last thrust, shaking as he came deep in her. Judging by her face and sudden silence, she finished as well.

Jared pulled himself out of her and turned to me. "I'm not done with you yet," he told me with a sound that told me that he was serious. He leaned over me, towering over my small body. He grasped my breast and let his fingers return to my clit, gently grazing over the swollen little nub that was desperate for attention and release. My breathing got quicker as he touched me, and my hips thrust into him. I wanted him—bad. I pulled him against me, and he lowered his head to lick at my clit instead, first circling around it before finally flattening his tongue and pressing against it, rubbing and licking it until I couldn't take it any longer.

Just before I could get over the edge, he pulled away, leaving me ultimately disappointed as I looked up at him. He smirked. "Not so fast. I want to really enjoy my gift," he told me as he let his cock just barely touch the outside of my slit, driving me wild. I pushed up, hoping he'd give in, but he pulled back even further. He flipped me over onto my back and positioned me just right so that he could slam in from behind.

He thrust deeper and deeper into me, pushing further from behind. He was rubbing up against my inner walls. He pulled my head back, hooking my mouth with his fingers. I could taste myself on him, or maybe it was Becca on his fingers, either way, I let him pull me further and further back against him, letting myself get lost in the moment. I loved every moment of the fucking as his cock went deeper into me than I thought was possible.

"Do you like that?" he grunted as I moaned in ecstasy, pushing my ass up and slamming it against him to get him in me as deep as possible. I wanted him to fuck me harder.

"Yes," I gasped out between moans of pleasure. "Harder," I told him, and he obliged instantly. He let go of my head and slapped my ass, yanking my hair this time as he rode me. I felt him getting harder within me as he grew rougher. "Harder!" I cried out again.

He stopped and flipped me over again, looming over me, his cock ready for more action. He slapped at my thighs, leaving red welts on them before turning to slap me across the face. "I'll fuck your cunt harder," he told me as he thrust in deeper. I was in total ecstasy, feeling the waves of pleasure continue to rise up. He fucked and fucked until the lines between pain and pleasure were blurred, and I found myself succumbing to another wave of pleasure overcoming my whole body. I convulsed against his cock, once, twice, three times, and tightened up around him, moaning loudly. I could hardly think in the moment, and he pulled out.

"Done already?" He shoved his cock in my face. "Suck it."

I obliged, still trying to catch my breath. I sucked his cock into my mouth, tasting my cum all over it as my tongue slid down the shaft. I forced it down my throat deeply and sucked and sucked. I looked up at him and moaned against his cock, letting him feel my tongue near his head, and lingered on the frenulum. I lifted my hands to his cock and rubbed with them too, pulling down with my hands as I pulled my head and tongue back. I used the tip of my tongue to swirl around the head of his cock as I sucked, letting him hear my slurping.

He seemed to be loving it, as pretty soon, I could feel his hips starting to tense up. He wasn't going to last much longer. I watched him watching me and then reached over for Becca to get involved. I reached for her, beckoning her closer as I stopped sucking. I made space for her, and she quickly obliged, turning to lick his cock with me. We were on either side of his cock, sharing it as we licked, one at a time, on either side. I grabbed his balls, giving them a quick fondle and pressed against the perineum behind them, pushing up. His moans betrayed his pleasure and we could feel his cock starting to pulse against us harder. He was building up that fluid; he wouldn't last for much longer.

"How do you want to cum, birthday boy?" I purred for him, looking up with my best fuck-me eyes, and he smirked.

"On both of you," he said matter-of-factly between his breathing. His voice was low, husky, and sensual as he demanded it. He pushed against us with his cock, and we both started to lick at it again.

I sucked on his cock as Becca moved down for the balls, licking and sucking on them gently. We both kept going, feeling his cock swelling even more. He was just about to cum—we could both feel it as we tried to suck even more on him. It wouldn't be that much longer.

I felt his hand roughly grab the back of my hair, and I could see that he grabbed Becca as well, holding our heads steady as I kept sucking. His eyes were closed, head back as he thrust deeper and deeper into my mouth before he finally pulled himself out of my mouth, shifting to his hand.

He used his hand to keep jerking himself off, aiming his cock at both of us and finally, the strings of fluid came out of his cock, first on me and then onto her as well, spurting out in several streams as he groaned his pleasure, watching both of us as he did. He slowed to a stop after and looked at his handiwork. Both of our faces had strings of cum all over them, and the sight must have pleased him based on that satisfied smirk.

"Clean it off," he demanded, holding his cock to me, and I put the whole thing in my mouth, sucking and pressing my tongue against the bottom of his shaft to get the rest of that fluid out of him, swallowing it. "And each other, too," he told us.

I looked at Becca closer this time; she had it all across her lips and her cheek. Her tongue was already making quick work of the cum on her lips, but she couldn't reach on her cheek. I leaned forward and gently licked it away, letting my tongue linger as I did. When she was clean, she returned the favor, licking along my face as well. He chuckled to himself at the sight. "Good girls," he said huskily as he collapsed onto the bed, thoroughly spent.

"Happy birthday," we both told him as we curled up on either side of him without a care in the world. I didn't mind sharing with Becca at all, and in fact, it had actually been far more fun than I expected to share with her, and I wasn't quite sure that we'd never attempt that again. In fact, I would have loved to do that again in the future. It would be absolutely thrilling to get to fuck each other again, but not quite yet. I had had my fill. It was absolutely time for a nap before we decided on a round two.

Closer to the Edge

Erin is *frustrated*. She just wants a quiet home and a good, hard fuck that will leave her satisfied, and unfortunately, luck is not in her favor as she finds herself lacking both of those. She's woefully single with little desire to go out and find a one-night stand, and her neighbor loves to blast loud music to hide his own actions on a regular basis. Confronting her darkly sexy neighbor, Damian, to turn off his music, she finds herself tangled up in some sexy playtime that may be more than she ever bargained for, and she can't get enough of it.

I could hear the loud music pulsing against my wall in the apartment. It was loud and annoying, and I never wanted to hear that same bassline again. Of course, the neighbor never cared when I complained. I had tried telling him that his constant thundering about made it impossible for me to do my studying, and he laughed at me. I told him once that I couldn't sleep when he was listening to that loud music all night long and he told me to wear earplugs. When I tried telling him that he needed to learn to respect the people around him, he told me that all I needed was a good fuck because I was too uptight.

Now, I'll be honest; I hadn't had a good fuck in a while. But, that didn't mean that I couldn't think about things clearly. Besides, that's what my toys were for. I didn't need a dick to have a good time. And I clearly didn't need a dick to enjoy myself. I tried to ignore the music that was playing and went about my day. I couldn't read my book. I couldn't focus on the games that I was playing. I could even hear their music through my headphones, and no matter how hard I tried, I couldn't get away from it.

I tossed and turned around in my bed, desperate for some sort of relief; I couldn't get away from the noise, and eventually, I had had enough! I took my robe, tied it up around me, and stormed over to his door. I pounded on it and waited. Of course, no response. The neighbor had given up answering the door to me long ago, no matter how much I tried to knock. I ended up pounding again.

"DAMN IT, DAMIAN OPEN THIS DOOR RIGHT NOW!!" I shouted, slamming my fists against the door. "I'VE HAD ENOUGH WITH THIS MUSIC ALREADY! TURN IT OFF AND GET OUT HERE!"

I raised my fist to slam against the door again, but as I swung, he finally opened the door, and my hand connected with his chest. He stood there with a cocky grin on his face, one eyebrow, pierced, raised up, and arms crossed in front of him.

"Can I help you, Erin?"

I stared at him in shock. I hadn't expected him to open the door—and yet here we were. He was looking right at me, face to face, and I couldn't figure out what to do next.

"Erin." He repeated himself. "Please take your hand off of me."

I realized that my fist was still against his chest and pulled away, embarrassed. "S-sorry. But seriously, Damian! I can't think with your music so loud! What is wrong with you?!"

"Nothing's wrong with me; I'm just having a good time. It sounds like you need some practice learning about what a good time means," he replied. He held the door open wider, inviting me in, and I hesitated, not totally convinced that I wanted to enter.

Damian was the stereotypical bad boy neighbor. He wore all black, and his current tank top was skin-tight and taut, revealing the abs underneath. He wasn't a bad guy—I knew that much. I saw him occasionally carrying up groceries for the elderly neighbors and saw him feeding a stray cat outside once. But, he was also highly annoying. He lived in a corner unit, and I had the only unit that connected to his, so lucky me, I got to hear all of his music in all of its annoying blaring that I desperately wished I could make go away.

"Don't be a buzzkill, Erin. Get in here," he told me with that trademark smirk.

I huffed but finally went in. Why not? Maybe, if I talked to him like a normal human being, he'd actually shut up and let me live in peace.

We went into his home, and thankfully, he *finally* turned down the music to a tolerable level. It was still annoying, but at least it was no longer unbearable as the bassline continued heavily, punctuated by all sorts of drums. I had never been in his home before, and looking around, I could see why. It was clean, but at the same time, I had not been prepared to see what was in there.

The living room was lined with sex objects. There was no shortage of beads and dildos lining up and down the walls, and there was what appeared to be a bunch of restraints in there as well. I looked around at everything and turned to look at Damian with a look of mortification on my face. He must have caught onto it because he smirked at me. "Problem?" he asked.

"N-no..." I managed to squeak out, feeling my face flush. I looked around for somewhere to sit, unsure I really wanted to sit down in the first place. Did I really want to touch anything in here?

"Do you like what you see?" His voice had a hint of edge to it, and he looked at me with that look I hadn't seen from someone in a long while. It was the look of someone wanting to consume what was in front of them. He was loving every moment of this, and honestly? The sound of his voice kind of got me going almost immediately, and I suddenly became aware of the fact that I was really only wearing a robe with just my underwear underneath it and I flushed even brighter.

His cock was hard in his pants, and he didn't seem to care about it at all. He simply walked over to me to usher me to his couch and sat me down. I wasn't sure what I was thinking when I agreed to come in.

"So, Erin," he said, looking at me. He stood in front of me, and I was at eye level with his hard cock. "What is it that you came over here for?"

"Your music was too loud," I told him, trying hard not to look at his cock in my face. But, the harder I tried to resist from looking at him, the more that I really just wanted to. I was wet underneath my robe, and I prayed that he wouldn't be able to tell or smell it or anything else. I hoped that I'd be able to just sneak out and enjoy the rest of my quiet night.

"Really," he said, leaning in toward me. His face was right next to mine now as he leaned, and I could feel his breath on my skin. I wanted to slap him and kiss him all at the same time, and I could feel my clit at attention, ready for some loving that it had been so denied lately. It wanted to be touched. *I* wanted to be touched, but I didn't want him to know it.

"I can see how turned on you are right now," he whispered. "Your eyes... Your lips... I can smell it on you." He looked at my lips and bit his own, looking like he was ready to take them for his own. "You need to learn to lighten up, Erin," he purred to me. He looked at me closely, as if trying to discern my own interest. I could feel my own breath hitching as he looked at me, and I couldn't lie; the sexual tension was palpable between us. "I can teach you to lighten up."

"Really." I looked at him and scowled, crossing my arms in front of me.

"Yes, Erin, really," he told me. "Give it a shot. Besides, what's wrong with a little night of fun every now and then? Want a drink?"

I hesitated. Even though my mind wanted to say no, my body was begging me to give in. My body was begging for that connection and human touch. I needed it more than I have ever needed anything in my life, and I desperately wanted to accept in that moment. So I did something unexpected.

"Sure."

"Are you a wine kinda girl?" He looked me over as if trying to figure out my drink preference on his own.

"Whiskey, neat."

"Oho, big taste for someone so small, huh?" He smirked. "Coming right up."

He returned a few moments later with the drink in his hand and handed it over for me to sip at. I downed it, the whole two shots worth and handed him the cup back, proving the point. I wasn't some delicate flower, a special snowflake that wanted the world to cater to me. I just wanted some peace and quiet.

"So, Erin. Let's talk about boundaries."

"What kind of boundaries?" I glanced around his room and realized that we were in what was probably some sort of sex playroom, and suddenly, the loud music made sense. Was it there to drown out the sounds of fucking? That was honestly kind of hot, I realized, and my mind started to wander. Was every time the music got blasted a time when he was getting fucked? Was it possible that he was just enjoying the moment, or was he trying to hide the sounds of passion from me?

"What are you willing to do, and what are you not willing to do?"

"We'll get to that when we get to it!" I insisted, deciding to rush past that. I didn't want to talk about what I wanted and what I didn't.

"Fine, let's at least set up a safe word," he told me, and I started to worry a bit. Should I be concerned about what was going to happen? Safe words made it sound like it would be almost... violent. "Yellow for you're approaching a boundary. Red if you need to stop. I will respect those safe words. You can beg for me to stop, but unless you say, 'red,' I'm not stopping."

I nodded.

"Repeat the safe words to me, Erin."

"Yellow for slow down, red for stop."

"Very good," he replied. "Now, are you ready?"

"Yes." I looked at him and actually made eye contact without feeling feelings of rage for a moment. It was totally different than when we were fighting. I felt a strange mix of arousal, anticipation, and a bit of nervousness as well. What did the night have in store for me?

"Take off your clothes," he told me.

"That's rather forward, isn't it?"

Damian's hand wrapped around a flogger that he had in his back pocket, and he pulled it out. "I punish dirty little girls that don't listen to me," he purred, his eyes shining with arousal. He watched me closely, waiting to see if I said the safe words that we had talked about. I almost did, but I wanted to see where the night could go. Instead, I stripped as asked.

His eyes betrayed the surprise that I had only been wearing a bra and underwear underneath the robe, but he grinned at me, a dark, almost sadistic grin as he looked me over. "You've got quite the hot body, you little slut," he told me as his eyes rested on my breasts. "Take the underwear off, too. I want my toys to be completely naked. I'll be patient with you this time since you're new to being my little plaything, but I expect compliance."

Wordlessly, I started to drop the clothes onto the floor, and he suddenly swatted at me, making me squeal and pull my hand back in shock. I hadn't been expecting that. My hand, where I had been swatted, was already bright pink.

"You will respect me when I talk to you," he demanded. "You will say, 'yes, sir' when I tell you to do something. Do you understand?" His cock bulged and twitched in his pants.

"Yes, sir," I managed to say, rubbing my hand.

"Good. Now, strip."

"Yes, sir."

He tossed my clothes to the floor and inspected my completely naked body, nodding his approval. "Now, turn around. Bend over."

I was kind of shocked at the suddenness, but for some reason, I complied. "Yes, sir." When I bent over, he got to see my ass and lips in full view, and he chuckled to himself.

I couldn't see him, but I could feel his breath on my skin as he inspected my body. "It looks like you're already raring to go," Damian commented offhandedly, as matter-of-factly as you would expect someone to be over the weather. His finger traced the entrance of my pussy, picking up the liquid that I had already started to leak before sucking it off of himself. "This poor little pussy looks like it was neglected.

To be fair, it had been and hearing him say that only made me hotter for him. I felt my clit twitch, and he chuckled, putting his finger on it, rubbing it gently in soft circles that felt so good that I moaned. It had been so long since I had been touched by someone else that way. He continued to circle around it, watching my reaction as I sat there and let him have his way with me.

"Today's an exercise in patience, do you hear me?" he growled at me as he continued to rub along my clit. "If you are patient, you will be rewarded. If you get impatient or you're a naughty slut that can't control that sloppy pussy of yours, you will be punished. And trust me, I don't take my job lightly. I hand out punishments that I intend to keep."

"Yes, sir!" I squeaked as I felt his finger penetrate into my slit, stroking the inner walls. I felt the flogger that he had used on my hand dangle above my back, tickling and exciting the nerve endings in my bare skin as he did. The leather was cool and soft to the touch when it was not swung to sting, and it further excited me. I felt myself clench around his finger, and just as it did, he pulled his finger out from inside of me. "Slow down there, little slut. Enjoy the ride. You need a lesson in patience." He swatted my ass with the flogger, and I cried out as it stung against me. It had caught me off guard, but after the initial shock, it wasn't so bad after all.

"I'm sorry, sir," I gasped out. I didn't want to tell him the truth—that I was just a desperate, lusty slut that hadn't been fucked in far too long, so instead, I remained silent. I didn't say a word beyond that; I just looked over my shoulder, giving him the best fuck-me eyes I could.

He flipped me over and took my hand, leading me over to a bed, which he promptly pushed me onto. He was rough, but not hard enough to scare or worry me, and I went down as he wanted. He walked over to a drawer and pulled out a few different things, and when he came back, I saw this strange collar and a blindfold. I balked at the sight, and he hesitated for just a moment, giving me the chance to use those safe words if I wanted to, but when I didn't say a word after a few beats, he moved forward and got to work. He wrapped the restraint around me and before I knew it, my arms were tied to my neck and torso, and my legs were spread open. If I tried to move too much or if I tugged the leg restraints to put my legs back down, the restraint would tighten around my neck, forcing me to stay put, and the blindfold was added as well.

I couldn't see anything at all, but I could hear Damian moving around the room, and suddenly, there were headphones placed firmly over my ears, and the music was turned on. It was quieter music at the very least, but it was the same bass-heavy music that he normally listened to. I groaned my displeasure, but before I could remain irritated for long, I felt his cock at long last finally slide into my pussy and bring me that joy that I had been missing in my life. He slid right into me and I was shocked at how large he was. Holding my legs up at that angle actually made it better and the occasional tightening around my neck actually

elevated the sensations of being fucked as
Damian continued to go at it.

I felt myself starting to tense up, my poor,
neglected pussy too weak to resist the desire to
cum, and before I knew it, I was exploding with
pleasure. It must have been just four or five
thrusts before I had already finished, moaning
out loud and momentarily forgetting the order
that I had been given. As the orgasm ended, I
felt Damian's flog hit against my ass again,
stinging and making me yelp in pain. He drew
back and hit again and again, and I whimpered.
The music stopped suddenly as the headphones
were removed from my head. "You're in for a
punishment now, Erin. You were a selfish girl
and selfish girls get punished." And just as
suddenly as the headphones were removed,
they were replaced and the music was turned
up a notch or two, growing more intense.
I was a bit concerned when I realized that I
wasn't feeling anything at all. I couldn't feel
him moving around and obviously couldn't
hear or see him. It made me nervous, but there
was nothing that I could do, other than maybe
saying the safe word, but that would be
admitting that he won.

My legs were starting to burn with the effort to
keep them up, and I could feel them trembling.
I swear, Damian was laughing somewhere
nearby, even if I couldn't hear him, and
suddenly, I felt him approach. The air shifted
and I knew he was coming. I expected to feel

another lash of the whip, but instead, I was pleasantly surprised; a vibrator was placed against my clit, and it was happy to jump right back to action. I felt it stirring to life again, willing to go for a round two. It had been so long that I may as well enjoy it again. My clit twitched underneath the weight of the vibrator and I moaned, feeling my hips lift of their own accord as it rested against my body. I grinded against it, enjoying the moment, but just as I started to really get going, feeling my pussy starting to soak itself, I felt the vibrator disappear.

I gasped as it was pulled away, and instinctively, I looked around, only to be reminded that I couldn't see or hear anything. I sighed to myself. Was this my punishment? Was he just going to be a tease? At the very least, it would still be fun, I told myself.

Next, I felt his mouth on my nipple, going around the tip with his tongue gently and carefully, not willing to do anything too intense. He danced about my nipple, making me wetter than before. I moaned, my pussy feeling achingly empty, and there was nothing for me to push up against. I couldn't even clench my legs together to try to make myself feel better—all I had was waiting for him to come back to me and who knew when that would be? His tongue spun about my nipple again before letting go. He hovered just above it. I could feel his breath on the wet skin with every breath, driving me madder than before.

He moved to the other nipple then, but never quite touched it, keeping his lips tantalizingly above my skin so close that I could touch it, but not close enough to bring me to any sort of release. I could feel him, and it felt good, but it was making me desperate. My pussy was sopping wet now, and I could smell my fluids all throughout the room. I could feel the slight vibrations on the bed—he must have laughed at my expression of sheer indignation at the deprivation that I was facing.

Damian moved away; suddenly, the air was colder around me, and he left me there for a few minutes. All that I had to keep me company was the throbbing of the bass in the song, throbbing much like my swollen, tortured pussy that wanted to be filled up, and when I finally felt like I couldn't take it anymore, I felt his tongue on me. It was flat and hard as he pressed it against my clit, letting his tongue caress the little nub while his fingers danced just outside of my slit, greedily touching everything that they could.

He plunged his tongue into me, and I moaned, back arching as he did it. He was getting more and more creative with what he was doing to me, and he was making it perfectly clear that he had no intention of ever actually letting me get off. As I'd start to tense up again, he pulled back, just long enough for my aching, quivering pussy to slow down before starting up again. Just as he'd get a rhythm, sensing the impending release, he'd change it up completely, sending me crashing back down and needing to be worked up again.

I felt like crying with desperation as this continued. He shifted from his mouth to his cock for a while, fucking me deeply and hard, only to stop when he thought that I was getting too into it. He teased me silly, and the whole time, I couldn't do anything. I was at his utter mercy, and there was no way for me to do anything but sit there and take it and hope that maybe, he'd show just a bit of compassion and let me get off.

Of course, that never happened as he expertly played with my body like it was made just for him. Maybe it was with how well he was able to turn it on and keep it going—all I knew was that I wanted to fuck him silly, free of the restraints, but I knew that if I said the safe word, it would all be over.

He pulled out again, this time, squirting his load all over my chest as he did, leaving his sticky cum all over me as he licked it up, little by little off of me. He rubbed around my breasts, but never touched the nipples as he ran his hands over me. And finally, he lifted up the headphones, making it possible for me to hear his voice in my ear.

"You have something to be mad about now, you dirty slut," he whispered as he released the bonds and removed the blindfold.

I sat there in shock as I looked at him. He looked satisfied with himself as he looked at the massive puddle that I had left on his bed. He looked over me as I stared back at him, and he waited for me to do something.

"That's it?" I finally managed to say, frustrated.

"That's it," he confirmed. "Naughty girls aren't rewarded in this house. You didn't hold out for me, and you didn't get rewarded any further." He leaned over, planted a kiss atop my head, patted my frustrated pussy, and handed me my robe. "Don't worry, Erin, I'll keep the music down lower for you," he said with a wink as I picked up my clothes and put them on, in shock. As frustrated as I was, I had to admit that he had been the best lay I had had in a very long time. When I was ready to go, he held the door open politely. "I'll see you again very soon," he murmured as I walked by, smirking.

I scowled, both frustrated with the end result of our encounter and the fact that he was right— he *would* be seeing me again in the near future. There was no way I could resist that cock again, and I'd have to be more disciplined next time to actually enjoy it.

Shut Up and Fuck Me

Krissy is a secretary that often feels like she doesn't get appreciated enough. She hates when she is stuck working late on Fridays when she's waiting for her boss to finish working so she can wrap everything up, and so one day, she decides to spice things up. Horny and with nothing else to do while she waits for her boss, the CEO of a financial institution, to finish up, she fantasizes about fucking him, or rather, him fucking her, while she has some fun with herself. Is it possible that the fantasies could become a reality when he walks out to her with her fingers inside of her?

I closed the laptop in front of me and sighed to myself. I had all this work to do, but I only had one thing on my mind: Hard, thick cock. More specifically, hard, thick cock slamming into me over and over again to get me off. I was so wet and horny as I sat there at my desk. I was all alone in the office, save for my boss, Mr. Roberts, in the room behind a closed door. He didn't like to be bothered while he worked, and he was scheduled to be on a conference call for another twenty minutes or so. I sighed again, letting my hand slide over my arm as I did. I wanted that release—no, I *needed* that release, and I didn't know how I could expect to get it. I needed to find some way to release all of that pressure that had built up within me, but it seemed so indecent to do it at work, knowing that my boss could open the door at any point in time to ask me to do something.

But for some reason, the idea of him opening the door only made it seem hotter than before. The idea of getting caught actually made me hotter than anything else. I imagined the scenario out in my mind. I was touching myself, probing at my innermost bits and feeling my wetness, groping my breasts, hair askew, and nipples poking out of my shirt for easier access for my wandering hands. I was moaning to myself in joy, and the door opens. Instead of getting up or apologizing or trying to cover myself up, I would stare my boss in the eyes as I continued to finger fuck myself, giving him those eyes that would dare him to come over and get involved as well.

He would get involved in that scenario in my mind. He would be so overcome with desire at the sight of his secretary fucking herself that he would throw himself at her, putting her up on the table and fucking her silly. His cock, I imagined, would be long, hard and thick, and it would fill me up so much that I would worry that I would tear. His hands would be needy as they ran over my body, tugging desperately, and his breath would be heavy in my ear as he whispered into it that he wanted to fuck me more than anything else.

The image of him plunging himself into me over and over again was almost overwhelming.

I found myself gasping at the sight, and I realized that my fingers were wet—I had already slid down my skirt and was fingering myself. I glanced at his door—still locked, and I could hear his occasional roaring laugh as someone that he was trying to woo into a business deal said something that was probably not the least bit funny, but he laughed anyway in hopes that it would lighten the mood. I imagined the look on his face if he were to walk out right that moment—it would be shock and instant arousal as he did and I imagined the bulge in his pants that would grow as he did. It made me hotter to think about all of this, and I felt myself get even wetter as my fingers touched my insides. I rubbed against my inner wall almost lazily as my mind wandered.

What if instead, he threw me over the desk and fucked me silly from behind? His cock would be so hard and so satisfying as it pushed within me, deeper and deeper, as he demanded that I let him ravish my body, and I would not have a care in the world. I didn't care that we were at work and that he, or I, could lose a job over it. I imagined the sheer carnal pleasure at fucking someone without inhibitions, just enjoying each and every moment as it happened. I imagined the joy that I felt, letting him slam into me. It was so hot.

I felt myself let out a little whimper, biting my lip as I let my fingers dance around my clit. I felt myself feel a bit more desperate for that release, but I also didn't want it to end so quickly. I wanted to savor the moment. I wanted to live vicariously and dangerously, and right now, sexually explicit behaviors right in front of my boss's door seemed like a great way to make that happen. Maybe I was fucked up, I thought if I thought that the idea of potentially getting caught fingering myself was hot, but I didn't care, not in the moment.

My other hand reached over my breast, tantalizingly stroking the smooth skin. I reached down my shirt and let my fingers graze over my nipple. It felt so good as my nipple immediately responded, hardening underneath the touch. I licked my lips as I let my fingers trace the slit beneath the clit, but never entering me. Fuck, I needed to bring a vibrator to hide in my desk, or even in my purse, I told myself. It could be hot having someone find it in my desk, or having the security officer that has to check our bags make eye contact with me, blushing when he realizes that I'm carrying around a sex toy. It's not illegal, so he can't confiscate it, but he can think all about what I'm going to do with it later on.

I let myself tease myself a bit longer, running along the inner labia before I finally plunge my fingers in to rub at my inner walls. They are tight now from all of the buildup and tension that I have made as I continued to play with myself, and I looked over to the door. Still nothing, but he had to be getting close to wrapping up that business call now... and sure enough, I saw the light on the office phone turn off, signaling that he had hung up.

It was now or never, I told myself, looking at the door. Did I stop, or did I push my luck and see what would happen next? I decided to take my chances, drawn by the heady hormones coursing through my body and the feeling of excitement that was growing more and more tantalizing by the second the longer that I touched myself, and sure enough, I heard the click of the lock and the door handle opening up. I looked away from the door, throwing my head back in pleasure and pretending that I didn't see him coming out.

The door opened as I continued to finger fuck myself, and there was a moment of silence. I realized that touching myself was feeling even better, but it was not a cock in my vag—that's what I wanted more than anything else.

"Krissy?"

I heard his voice. It was bewildered at the sight. It was shocking, and possibly even a little turned on by the waver that I heard as if he was hesitant to stop me from the sexual release that I was so clearly enjoying. Head still tossed back in enjoyment; I opened my eyes to meet his gaze, slowly pulling my fingers out of my mouth and licking my fingers, one by one. I watched as his eyes widened slightly in response, but he never looked away. I could see his pants tighten, and I smirked. Instead of waiting for him, I stood up and walked toward him.

"I need you to fuck me right now," I told him in a low voice, looking at him through my eyelashes and pushing out my chest. One of my nipples was poking out for him to see, and I picked up his hand in my own, placing it on my chest. I pushed my hips against him, grinding on his rock-hard erection in his pants, and I pushed him toward his office without another word. He shockingly didn't fight back, considering that he was so much larger than I was. He seemed willing to comply with whatever I was going to ask him to do.

He probably thought that it was his lucky day; I told myself with a satisfied smirk as I felt the ache in my pussy grow more intense. I pushed him toward his chair. "I want you to do exactly what I say, do you understand me?" I told him without waiting for much of an answer as I pressed against his chest, urging him to sit down. He did, and I straddled him, rubbing myself against his cock that was still trapped in his pants. It was about as big as I had been hoping, I realized, and that was absolutely fitting for a man of his stature. I whined to myself as I felt his hardness underneath me and I grinded against it harder.

"I'm going to tie you up and have my way with you. I need your rock-hard cock in me so bad right now. You don't even know how badly I need to feel you within me," I told him, looking around for something—anything—that I could use to secure him behind me. I settled for some zip ties that I found in his drawer and put them on him, just behind the back of his chair. It wasn't much, but it would be enough for me to have my fun. A part of me was shocked that he was not protesting, but that only made it better in my book. I felt myself getting wetter, and I looked my boss over. He was the CEO of a major financial firm, and here I was, tying him up and getting ready to fuck both of our brains out, totally in control of every single moment of it.

Satisfied with how secure he was, I looked at his face. He was silent and watching me, but I could see the pleasure shining in his eyes. Did he get off on being dominated? I smirked, unzipping his pants and releasing his cock. It was still just as rock hard as it had felt inside of them as it sprang to attention, and I ran my fingers up and down over the length, enjoying the twitches that I got in response. He was turned on by that, too, it seemed. I chuckled to myself as I lowered my head onto his cock to suck on it. I didn't want to just throw myself onto him without first letting him warm up. He needed to be nice and ready, and the harder that he was, the better.

As I sucked on his cock, I heard him groan in pleasure, thrusting his cock closer to me as he did. He pushed up toward me, and I chuckled on his cock, letting my tongue linger as I let go of it. "Someone's ready for a good fuck," I purred as I looked up at him from his cock, my lips still touching it right around the frenulum as I spoke. His hips thrust forward as I did. "Aren't you going to say anything at all?" I asked him as I licked at his frenulum some more.

"You are fucking hot as hell," he managed to get out between heavy breaths. "I've wanted to get you over my desk ever since I hired you."

I laughed, rubbing over his cock. "Well, who's got whom now?" I asked as I took off my shirt, revealing my toned stomach and perky, D-cup breasts. I lowered them around his cock, letting him rub it between the soft, warm skin as I held them together and kneaded at my nipples for even more pleasure than before. I loved every moment of what I was doing, and from the look on Mr. Roberts' face, he did too.

I felt his dick getting harder as I rubbed him down with my breasts. "Oh, Mr. Roberts," I moaned, looking up at him, "Don't cum already. I've got so much more in store for you than this." Just saying that as I rubbed my tits over him got him cumming, and he squirted all over my tits and my face.

He seemed almost embarrassed that he had cum already, but he didn't say a word.

"Uh, oh, someone made a mess," I purred, using my finger to clean up every last drop of cum from my skin and licking it up, enjoying the taste in my mouth. I leaned forward to suck the last of it from his cock, too. There was no use in wasting the good stuff when I was right there and more than willing to suck it up if there was nowhere else to put it. I licked it up and looked at him with a smirk. He was watching me in awe, as if he had never seen someone do that before. His cock stayed mostly hard, even after he had spilled so much. As it started to soften, I sucked on it and licked at it, trying to keep the blood flow there. I rubbed myself on it, getting back onto his lap and straddling him. I removed my panties and left the skirt on, letting myself rub up on him over and over to bring him back to life. I put my tits in his face for him, letting them bounce with every motion that I made to try to wake his softening dick up again for more.

He leaned over and took control then. He sucked on my left tit first, licking desperately at it and then finally pulling the whole thing into his mouth, his tongue spinning all around it as he did. He was rough, but not hurtful as he tugged at my nipples. He licked and sucked on them carefully, and the more that I rubbed on him, the closer to finishing that I got. I couldn't hold out for much longer, I realized. I needed to fuck him soon, or I wouldn't be satisfied, but his cock was still woefully unready for that.

Instead, I chose to let myself grind on him longer, waiting for that refractory period to end. I lost myself in the moment, rubbing the tip of his cock against my clit and letting his shaft rub up against the lips. Up and down, up and down I went, and I used my other hand to play with my other nipple as well. I lost myself in my mind again, imagining what would happen if I were to undo his ties right that moment. Would he bend me over? Would he fuck me raw? What would he do for me? I wanted to know.

I imagined him taking me from behind, his cock reaching the deepest part of me while his balls slapped at my clit with every thrust, fucking me to the best climax that I had ever felt. I imagined him flipping me over and fucking me silly on my back, his hands on my breasts and mouth on mine as he fucked harder and harder. His cock was large enough to make that happen; I had to admit that much. It looked like it would be exactly what I needed to finish myself off that night. All I needed to do was get it back to hard again.

I rubbed harder against it, desperation in my aching pussy apparent as I did it more and more. I felt him finally starting to respond, and as his dick swelled against me, I came atop him. My whole body betrayed me, with me rubbing harder and harder against him as my hips gyrated atop his own as I did.

He chuckled at me as he continued to suck on my tit. "Someone's enjoying themselves," he murmured, the sensation of his lips moving making me realize that even after a spectacular orgasm, I wanted *more*. I wanted to be selfish.

"You're going to fuck me," I told him, getting off of his lap and clipping the zip ties off of him so that he could get up. He rubbed his wrists as he regarded me with lust shining in his eyes and dick, pointing at the ready to keep going.

"I can do that," he replied, his hands suddenly on my hips as he turned me around and bent me onto his desk, sending items clattering to the ground. Neither of us paid any attention to it as we did, and I felt his hand on the back of my head, pushing it down and then shifting to my hips to line himself up just right. "I'll fuck you so hard that you won't be able to walk those pretty little legs out of here," he growled in my ear before he thrust into me.

He wasn't kidding. And I was all the happier for it. I wanted a good, hard fuck, and if he was willing to give it to me, I was happy. After all, all I had wanted was a hard cock inside of me one way or another.

I felt him thrust so deeply into me that I let out a guttural moan of pleasure, my back arching on its own accord as he did. He let his cock linger there inside of me, letting me finally enjoy what I had wanted more than anything. He let me clench against it tightly as he lingered there, and I was happy to do so. I clenched all around it over and over again, letting myself enjoy it.

Slowly, he pulled his rock hard cock out of me, and I tightened up again as if I could prevent it from leaving if I tightened up enough. It slipped out, leaving just the tip keeping my lips apart so that he would be able to thrust in again when he was ready. He let it rub against me, moving his hips in a circle to tease those sensitive, swollen, needy lips of mine, and it was driving me *crazy*. I wanted that cock back inside of me so bad.

I wanted it so bad that I shoved my ass toward him, plunging his cock right back into me without him being able to protest. I rode it harder on my own this time. I fucked it standing up, pushing myself onto him over and over again. His cock felt so good to ride as it glided in and out of my wet pussy, and I needed it so bad.

I pulled away and turned around to face him, pushing him to the floor. He obliged, laying across the thin carpet as I had requested, and I straddled him, preparing to ride him as hard and long as I wanted to. I pushed myself around him, letting his cock deepen, pushing my whole weight down to sit on him as I moaned in pleasure.

He reached around to play with my ass, placing his hands on either cheek before he started to guide my movements. He pushed up and pulled me back down to his own rhythm, and I was more than willing to oblige as we did. I felt myself getting hotter and tighter around him. His mound of fur around his cock was glistening with my juices and the smell of sex, hot and heady, filled the room as we fucked harder and with reckless abandon. I rode him gleefully, head tilted back as I did. I bounced harder on his cock, letting it get deeper and deeper into me as I did. I put his hands on my boobs to hold them in place as I looked into his eyes. He was watching me with an impressed, turned on expression as he rode me harder and harder. He wanted to fuck me just as much as I needed him, it seemed.

He let me have my fun before flipping me over, pulling my hair as he thrust deeper into me. He had one hair in my hair and another clawing at my chest, clenching down on my breasts tightly. His nails dug into my skin, just hard enough to avoid breaking the skin. He left his hands there, smashing his palm into my nipple and teasing me harder.

"It's my turn to do the fucking and the leading," he whispered in my ear. "And I want you to be a good girl and cum when I tell you to. Do you understand me?" His voice was breathy in my ear as he spoke, slamming into me as hard as he could.

I could barely speak as the pleasure began to build up again, and I nodded my head to him.

"Good girl. Now I'm going to ride your little ass hard until you cum when I tell you to." He wasn't joking, either. He fucked me so hard that all of the fantasies that I had been having, all of the visualization that I had been doing, was gone. He fucked me so hard that all I could focus on was the feeling of his cock inside of me, ramming me harder and harder.

He stopped suddenly, and I gasped at the sudden lack of sensation, suddenly flipping me over.

"I thought you were going to ride me?" I asked between heavy breaths with a smart ass smirk on my face.

"Oh, I will. But we're going to do something else first. He laid down on the floor and pushed my head toward his cock, soaked with my moisture. "Lick it."

I obliged, tasting the sex on his skin with a long moan of pleasure. It was so hot to taste our fluids combining. He pulled me closer and positioned me just above his face, and suddenly, I felt his tongue on me as well. He was tonguing me as I blew him, and I moaned on his cock again. I kept my grip on him tight. I could see that his balls were starting to tighten up, and I could feel the tension in his cock the more that I sucked him off, and I knew that if I kept it up, I'd be able to get him to cum.

But more importantly, he was licking me so much that I wasn't sure that I'd be able to hold out. His tongue skated across the tip of my clit as he slammed a finger into my pussy, reaching for the g-spot as he tongued me, and the feeling was so intense that I almost came right then and there. I was getting desperate as my poor, aching, soaking pussy craved to be filled up, and I stood up suddenly as I felt myself approaching the point of no return. I slipped past the grip he tried to use to hold me in place, and I got on his cock as quickly as I could, letting the pleasure build up even more until I could no longer take it. With a cry out that would make anyone blush, if they heard it, I came on that hard cock just as I felt him thrust up into me. We both moaned in pleasure, enjoying the ecstasy of each other's bodies as we came, our bodies spasming to each other in almost perfect harmony as we both finally got the big moment.

It felt like it went on for ages as my body, desperate for that release, clenched against him again and again until finally, spent and exhausted, I collapsed against his chest, sweaty, breathing heavily, and hearing his heart thundering against my ear. We weren't going to cuddle, but I took the moment to enjoy myself before getting up and straightening myself out. I cleaned myself up, taking a moment to glance in the mirror to see that I was looking quite disheveled.

Wordlessly, I put my clothes on and tried to make my appearance as appropriate to going out into the real world as I could. When I was satisfied, I turned to look at Mr. Roberts for a moment. He was reclining back in his chair, arms behind his head and looking fully satisfied himself as if it were not just his cock that had been stroked, but his ego as well. "I'll see you Monday, Krissy," he said with a smirk and a knowing look that said that this would probably become a regular thing.

I smirked right back at him as well. "See you on Monday," I replied cheerfully with a wave as I left, fully aware that my walking was not quite right. It seemed he had kept that promise after all.

Description

Warning: This book is for adults that are looking for something to drive them wild.

Are you looking for something to spice up your night? Look no further—this book features seven highly erotic stories that will tickle your fancy while you tickle something else. If you're into taboo, sexy stories filled with subjects that would make your mother blush, you're in the right place. Open this book and find something to get your panties soaked today. You'll find stories that are rough and sensual at the same time, tickling taboo fancies and wetting panties, such as:

- **Blind Pleasure:** A woman exploring a swinger's club with her husband getting a night that she'll remember forever after the sexy, sensual experience that she has with more than one man. Who knew so many different hands could feel so good?
- **Variety is the Spice of Sex:** A woman who is bored with her married sex life decides to bring in some reinforcements to relive her days of not being beholden to just one body, spending some sexy, sensual time with both her husband and their neighbor to spice their bedroom life up a bit more than they realized they needed. Variety is the spice of life—and sex!

- **Clara's Experiment:** A woman exploring her interest in being submissive learning what it really means to be bound and used like a toy for the thrill of someone else, being truly at the mercy of someone else, and discovers that she loves every single moment of it.
- **Amelia's Punishment:** A young, hot housekeeper makes a mistake that deserves to be punished. After all, what good is it to have housekeepers that can't do what they're told when they're told to do it? Sometimes, you need a firm hand to teach you what needs to be done, and her boss is not afraid to teach that lesson if he has to. In fact, he's more than willing to and teaches her a lesson she'll never forget.
- **Unwrapped Gifts:** If gifts are meant to be opened, does that mean that our clothes are just gift wraps for when we give ourselves to someone else? In this story, a woman and her best friend present themselves as the ultimate gift to her boyfriend for a celebration of a lifetime.
- **Closer to the Edge:** Noisy neighbors can be the worst—but what if they're also smoking hot and you're desperate? This story takes you alongside a woman who confronts her noisy neighbor, only to be in for a night that she'll never forget. Let's just say he gave her something to really be frustrated about.

- **Shut up and F*ck me:** Sometimes, when you have the urge, you have to satisfy it, and this hot secretary knows that better than anyone else. But, she wants to take things one step further and make her fantasies a reality when she knows that her boss is in the room next door, finishing up a business call. Can she convince him to give her what she wants?

www.ingramcontent.com/pod-product-compliance
Lightning Source LLC
Chambersburg PA
CBHW050735030426
42336CB00012B/1571